WINNING THE WELLNESS GAME

LAWRENCE POWER M.D.

TO

LUCY   MEMORY

Who Saved The Last Dance For Me

HEALTH
&
WELLNESS
PUBLISHING
AND
PROGRAMS
FOR OVER
TWO DECADES

WINNING
THE
WELLNESS
GAME

YOUR
PLAY BY PLAY
GUIDE
TO FULL HEALTH AND
PEAK PERFORMANCE

NATIONAL
HEALTH
SYSTEMS

LAWRENCE
POWER
M.D.

WINNING THE
WELLNESS GAME

By: Lawrence Power, M.D.
Published By: National Health Systems Inc.
26631 Southfield Road
Southfield, MI 48076

Copyright © 1991 Lawrence Power, M.D.
Library of Congress Catalog Number: 91-60284

ISBN 1-879963-04-3

PUBLISHER'S FORWARD

This book has been designed to help you, the reader, help yourself. It is sold with the understanding that the author is not engaged in rendering personal medical advice or professional service in this book.

It is not intended to trivialize the risks of serious disease, nor to deny that heart disease and blood pressure and obesity and cancer require professional intervention as early as possible. Every effort has been made to document opinions and to minimize mistakes, whether typographical or instructional. We recommend that you share any information contained herein with your personal physician. Many will be pleased to be made aware of the existence of this book.

Active patient participation is at the heart of the best outcomes with today's major illnesses. Self-care does not mean avoiding doctors or denigrating technology. It means becoming an informed participant in all processes. Neither the author nor the publisher can take responsibility for changes in your medical and dietary program. Self-care is neither self-diagnosis nor self-treatment, which are always potentially hazardous. Self-care is taking an active personal part in your own health under the supervision of a doctor sympathetic to the idea of preventive interventions. This is not a self-diagnosis or self-treatment book. It is a book to help your doctor help you help yourself.

A CAUTIONARY TALE

THE BEST HEALTH CARE IS SELF CARE

A recent patient of mine had learned of her high blood pressure at age 40, and after a number of rare diseases that can cause high blood pressure were ruled out by her physician, the commonest kind was ruled in. She had "essential hypertension". It's a name that means we really don't know what causes it, but it's the most common kind of high blood pressure. Salt plays a part, so she was discharged from her work-up in hospital on a daily water pill and a low salt diet.

The woman had a weight problem too, and was advised to lose at least 30 pounds. But she'd been overweight for years without high blood pressure, so she and her physician focused their attention on the pills for her pressure. She was seen in his office every three months where her pressure was judged to be "controlled" although her weight continued to rise. Diabetes developed while on the water pills when she was 46. This time, after a week in the hospital, she received further dietary advice--including the need to lose weight. But she'd been overweight for years without diabetes or blood pressure so another pill was added to bring her blood sugar under control. More visits, more pills, more weight gain. Its not an unusual experience or story.

She was 50 when she had a heart attack and spent several weeks recovering. But now, after discharge from hospital, she had pain in her chest when exerting herself. It was the heart pain called angina and, still overweight, she underwent coronary artery bypass surgery.

Throughout her 15 year medical odyssey, she remained heavy. It ran in the family, and she chose to accept it. But what runs in families these days, are tendencies more often than diseases themselves. The tendency to be overweight is a genetic predisposition that requires abundance to express itself. An abundance of food and an abundance of ease.

Beyond the relief of recovering from the procedure, the bypass surgery was a disappointment, as is usually the case. It failed to relieve her breathlessness or fatigue, so she finally faced the problem of her weight. Over a period of six months, and supervised by a new physician, she shed 43 excess pounds and was transformed. The diabetes disappeared. The high blood pressure disappeared. She no longer needed medication and she was no longer tired or breathless. In fact, she was cured or, more correctly, she came under biological control.

She's now in her mid-50s, back on the job and off all medication. She walks briskly for an hour every day. Her health insurance company had paid out more than $40,000 on her behalf, but refused to reimburse for the costs of controlling her weight. Lots for the treatment, naught for the cure.

ACKNOWLEDGEMENTS

The practice of medicine is changing, in part because of technical progress and in part because our perception of disease is changing. This book is an acknowledgement of trends that are only now, in the 1990's, getting well under way.

The author has been fortunate to have spent the first half of his professional life in a variety of clinical centers in several countries around the world, getting involved in the care of literally tens of thousands of patients. This experience has lead to the conviction that most of us in the developed world are suffering to some extent from self-inflicted wounds.

Over the years, dozens of individuals as teachers, colleagues, patients or researchers have contributed to the conclusions that motivated the production of this book. To all of them, the author's debt is total. But the most important contributors have been those patients who provided the privilege of their confidence and the opportunity of their insights.

ABOUT THE AUTHOR

Dr. Lawrence Power was trained in endocrinology at the University of Michigan, and is a practicing physician in Detroit, Michigan. His academic credentials include professorships at the University of Michigan and at Wayne State University, but it was his years as Chief of Medicine at Detroit General Hospital that had the most profound influence on his thinking and his career:

"Over the years, watching the steady readmission of previously discharged patients was a constant reminder of how short-lived were the successes of our earlier efforts. The majority of our patients had diseases of personal mismanagement and I came to the realization that real health and a greater sense of professional satisfaction would more likely come from teaching patients the more durable strategies of self-care."

In 1980, Dr. Power established his own Lifestyle Clinic in Southfield, Michigan. Devoted to teaching patients the science of self-care, it is a clinic like few others...from state of the art diagnostic evaluation, to fitness and food preparation. Programs offered at the clinic have formed the basis of seminars undertaken at all of Detroit's auto companies as well as at businesses and for organizations throughout the state.

WINNING THE WELLNESS GAME is Dr. Power's health manifesto to the general public from this decade of daily experience. In vivid prose and with lively graphic assists, he guides the reader through contemporary mine fields of destructive habits to others giving greater promise of total health and full performance. As with his clinic, Dr. Power's health book is like no other.

A DISCLAIMER

SELF CARE IS NOT SOLO CARE

Work with your own physician as you work with this book. The ideal patient-physician relationship in the game of risk factor reduction is a player-coach relationship. No book on health care, however credentialled the author, can take the place of on-the-spot counsel from a professional who knows you and your situation from hands on contact.

Check first with your doctor regarding any food or fitness practice you propose to undertake to enhance your health. The author, as an author, is not engaged in the practice of rendering a medical service. That is the function of your personal health care provider. Self care is not solo care.

Every effort has been made to make this workbook useful and as accurate as possible. There may, however, be mistakes or positions that will change. Scientific findings, especially clinical scientific findings, are always provisional. There is always room for more testing, for new data, and a shift in emphasis or conclusions. Science is an unfinished business as is the game of wellness, so no book can ever be the last word. Talk to your doctor first.

ABOUT ADAPTIVE FAILURE

Life is a restless process, yet it craves the steady state. Changes that occur from minute to minute as part of daily living, continually threaten the steady state, forcing corrective adjustments, whether the threats are to our sense of balance, our blood pressure, temperature or peace of mind.

The most pervasive threat to the steady state of our health in this century, has been abundance, the abundance of food and the abundance of ease. We are creatures that emerged in scarcity and have learned that we handle abundance badly. To our surprise (and dismay), abundance can eventually lead to heart attacks, cancer, hypertension and diabetes, and the premature loss of 2 to 3 decades of life.

Adaptive failure results when the overloads of abundance cannot be accommodated, when the ideal or normal steady state cannot be preserved: The weight goes up, or the blood pressure, or the cholesterol and so on. Adaptive failure results from an interaction of your environment with your genes. Life indeed, is not fair. On identical diets, some people have a cholesterol problem or a weight problem or a blood pressure problem or a cancer problem, while others do not. Adaptive failure is the way this book looks at today's health risk factors because that takes you out of the passenger's seat and puts you into the driver's seat, or out of the stands and onto the playing field.

ABOUT THIS BOOK

Because the face you see in the mirror each day changes so little from year to year, it's easy to assume that your body is stable and set. Nothing, however, could be further from reality. Life is a process of change; constant, relentless, continuous change. Every cell in every tissue of the body is always in a state of dismantling, replacing, repairing and reassembling component parts.

Environmental concerns in recent years have made us all aware of food chains, how bigger creatures eat smaller creatures, to get the goods they need. But they are also getting an increasing assortment of bads. By paying greater attention to the goods and bads in our own lives, we can begin to help our tissues in their daily needs for replacement and repair

A total health tool kit has been assembled between the covers of this book to help you increase the goods and reduce the bads. Its an instructive guide to two major sets of health habits, with a unique self-paced scoring system to track your progress. Winning the Wellness Game is the complete risk factor reduction workbook.

COMMENTS

"Interesting, informative, and so practical it changed many of my attitudes and habits for the better..."

C.K., Elementary School Principal

"Only wish I'd known this stuff years ago when my family was younger..."

D.W., Homemaker

"Compelling information, clearly presented in a useful way."

W.T., Automotive Executive

"Liked the easy ways to remember important points. It was instructive and funny, in a practical package."

P.B., Social Worker

CONTENTS

PART ONE

THE GAME OF WELLNESS
An overview of where we are healthwise
and some of the ways we got there.

WHOLE FOOD FUNDAMENTALS

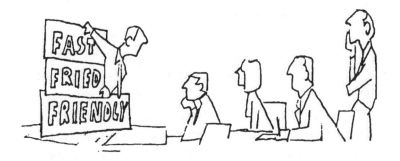

WHAT'S WRONG WITH THE BEST DIET IN THE WORLD?

T he Basic Four approach to a healthful diet is enshrined in nutrition teaching. It's a kind of shorthand that advises us to eat from four food groups every day for nutrition balance. There's a dairy group, a meat group, a fruit and vegetable group and a grain group. It's an approach to food, however, that can make you very sick.

It can send the blood pressure up with its potential load of

5

salt, and cause strokes. It can send the blood cholesterol up with its load of fat and cholesterol, and cause heart attacks. And much new evidence indicates that it can promote cancer. It's a nutrition guide whose time has gone. Not enough to convince you to rethink it all? Well, it can provide an intake of food so bereft of fiber that it leads to diverticulitis or appendicitis.

Back when the Basic Four was formulated, when it became our official food message, nutritionists were most concerned about deficiencies. They wanted us to get an adequate daily intake of calories, protein, calcium and vitamins. An apple a day kept the doctor away and we walked to work and worked 10-12 hours when we got there. Household chores took 16 hours a day, every day. Heart attacks were rare, and a glance at old photographs of crowds and celebrating groups reveals the extent of the changes since then in body sizes.The old concerns for getting enough have pretty well vanished. Iron deficiency is still around, as is calcium deficiency in older women but neither of these issues will benefit from more of the Basic Four, without worse consequences. Since the 1940s, advances in the science of food processing have made it very difficult to teach healthful food selections by referring to the Basic Four.

*"THE RULE OF HOLES SAYS THAT WHEN
YOU'RE IN ONE IT'S NOT SMART TO KEEP
DIGGING. AND WE'RE IN ONE."*

The Basic Four Food Groups lock us into a time warp which ignores two developments: Over 50 years of technical advances in processing that are more concerned with taste and appearance and shelf life than with nutrition and health and 30 years of scientific studies that have tied today's diseases to today's diet.

New food groupings are being proposed for the 1990s by appropriate national committees, but it's not an easy undertaking. So entrenched are the forces benefiting from our present diet that advisory boards specifically drawn up to recommend new national food policies have been repeatedly frustrated, aborted or paralyzed, producing a golden silence for the status quo.

In going down this road we've sacrificed the variety that once justified the Basic Four as a guide to balanced eating. An onion is nutritionally different from an apple and if both were eaten raw or steamed or baked, their nutrition differences and contributions would hold. But any differences between the two foods shrink to insignificance when they're eaten as onion rings or apple fritters. Taste good they do, but sick they are making us and costing plenty in terms of productivity, premature debility and medical dollars. No country in the world spends more on medical care. . . sorry, "health care," than we do, yet the citizens of many countries outlive us and "outwell" us. Life expectancy of American men is 19th among all nations; and for women 14th among other countries. Those outliving us eat differently.

We're not getting our money's worth nutritionally or medically by emphasizing so technical an approach to food and health, and by ignoring the advantages enjoyed around the globe through different lifestyles. The Rule of Holes says that when you're in one it's not smart to keep digging. And we're in one. More money is not the answer. New food and fitness practices are best and will be for the rest of this century.

No longer do we live in an age of simple food and simple effort. The need for physical exertion in our work-a-day world has been reduced to insignificance, and the food available to us is delicious. How comfortable, pleasant, and in many ways how welcome are these trends, but they have proven to be health undermining.

Without a correction of some of our current food excesses, sad to say, and without restoration of regular physical activity to our daily lives, we are pursuing a wandering trail of ill-health in the making. Mounting scientific evidence supports the position that change is needed. Only a few simple changes in food and fitness habits would add quality to our days and about a decade of energetic length to our lives.

IGNORE YOUR HEALTH LONG ENOUGH AND EVENTUALLY IT GOES AWAY.

MEET A HEALTH HABITS SCORECARD

On the next page you can see some food and fitness activities grouped into categories to create a score card. It is designed to help you begin tracking some good health habits. Let's look it over.

WHOLE FOOD HABITS are important to full health because they provide essential vitamins and minerals.

ADDITIONAL FIBER HABITS help overcome today's excessive refinement. We eat a third of the fiber we need.

LAXATION HABITS are an important indicator of digestive health. A normal stool is soft and formed and long and passed nearly every day.

AEROBIC FITNESS HABITS are essential to full performance as well as energetic longevity.

RECREATION HABITS are important because, as the word implies, they re-create. We are brain and body creatures who require brain and body variety in our lives.

Give each category some thought before entering your number. A completed ScoreCard on the next page can help serve as your guide to scoring.

YOUR STARTING SCORECARD™

1. RUNNING ALL THE BASES

SCORING: DAILY: 10   WEEKLY: 5   MONTHLY: 0
(MORE OR LESS) (TWICE OR THRICE) (SELDOM OR NEVER)

		You	Ideal
	WHOLE FOOD HABITS	SCORING	
FIRST BASE	FRESH / FROZEN / CANNED FRUITS:		10
	FRESH / FROZEN / CANNED VEGETABLES:		10
	WHOLE GRAIN BREADS / ROLLS / CEREALS / PASTAS:		10
	ADDITIONAL FIBER HABITS		
SECOND BASE	BEANS / PEAS / LENTILS:		10
	MUFFINS / BRANS / FIBERED CEREALS:		10
	FIBER SUPPLEMENTS-LAXATIVES / NUTS & SEEDS:		10
	LAXATION HABITS		
THIRD BASE	STOOLS: SOFT, FORMED & BUOYANT:		10
	PASSAGE: PAINLESS & BLOODLESS:		10
	AEROBIC FITNESS HABITS		
	BRISK WALKING, DANCING, RUNNING:		10
	TREADMILLING, AEROBICS, OTHER ACTIVITIES:		10
	RECREATION HABITS		
HOME PLATE	GARDENING, GOLFING, SWIMMING, OTHER:		10
	READING, HOBBYING, CONCERT-GOING, OTHER:		10

IF YOUR BASE-RUNNING IS:
ABOVE 100: FANTASTIC! KEEP IT UP
BETWEEN 75 AND 100:
  (YOU'RE ABOVE AVERAGE)
BELOW 50: YOU NEED A LITTLE R&R
  (REPAIR & RESTORATION)

Now add up all the scores from your habits.

YOUR BASE-RUNNING SCORE: | 120

MARTIN K RUNS THE BASES

A patient of mine has offered us a look at his own scorecard from an early office visit. He was a sedentary man of 45 years and on the facing page you see the results of his first self-assessment. His habits were typically those of a middle level, suburban living, automobile executive.

With WHOLE FOOD HABITS, he hesitated but then decided that his salads and canned vegetable intakes allowed him to score himself 10 points.

The only way he could score anything in the ADDITIONAL FIBER HABITS category was to count the mixed nuts he sometimes had with a pre-dinner drink.

LAXATION HABITS he puzzled over until they were explained as in Chapter 3.

By the time he got to AEROBIC FITNESS HABITS, the accumulating low scores disturbed him, so he entered "Golf" ... then checked the definition of aerobic.

In the RECREATION HABITS category, television gets the single largest chunk of his leisure time, but we let his scoring stand.

YOUR STARTING ScoreCARD™

MARTIN K

1. RUNNING ALL THE BASES

SCORING: DAILY: 10   WEEKLY: 5   MONTHLY: 0
(MORE OR LESS)   (TWICE OR THRICE)   (SELDOM OR NEVER)

		You	Ideal
	WHOLE FOOD HABITS	*SCORING*	
FIRST BASE	FRESH / FROZEN / CANNED FRUITS:	0	10
	FRESH / FROZEN / CANNED VEGETABLES:	10	10
	WHOLE GRAIN BREADS / ROLLS / CEREALS / PASTAS:	0	10
	ADDITIONAL FIBER HABITS		
SECOND BASE	BEANS / PEAS / LENTILS:	0	10
	MUFFINS / BRANS / FIBERED CEREALS:	0	10
	FIBER SUPPLEMENTS-LAXATIVES / NUTS & SEEDS:	5	10
	LAXATION HABITS		
THIRD BASE	STOOLS: SOFT, FORMED & BUOYANT:	0	10
	PASSAGE: PAINLESS & BLOODLESS:	10	10
	AEROBIC FITNESS HABITS		
	BRISK WALKING, DANCING, RUNNING:	0	10
	TREADMILLING, AEROBICS, OTHER ACTIVITIES: *golf*	0	10
	RECREATION HABITS		
HOME PLATE	GARDENING, GOLFING, SWIMMING, OTHER:	5	10
	READING, HOBBYING, CONCERT-GOING, OTHER:	10	10

IF YOUR BASE-RUNNING IS:
ABOVE 100: FANTASTIC! KEEP IT UP
BETWEEN 75 AND 100:
   (YOU'RE ABOVE AVERAGE)

BELOW 50: YOU NEED A LITTLE R&R
   (REPAIR & RESTORATION)

any score your honesty? add up all the scores from your habits.

YOUR BASE-RUNNING SCORE: 40 | 120

MARTIN K'S REACTION

Discouraged would be a fair description, and sobered. But he was the kind of individual who accepted challenge, who recognized the need to change for a better outcome.

Not to worry! Onward and upward he concluded, at least this scoring system will lead me in a direction I want. Stop the drift. Get to work on a few new Good Habits.

Now about the Bad Habits and my need to change a few of those too, well that's the other half of the wellness equation and the Habits ScoreCard...

FITNESS FEEDINGS

NIBBLING FOR THIN

Eat a piece of fruit for breakfast.

Keep some tiny boxes of raisins in your desk or car or purse.

Snack before you go anywhere - whether a cross-country drive, dinner out, a party, or a business meeting.

Take food with you when you go anywhere - to a movie, the beach, or the park.

Canned fruits and vegetables make good storage form food encounters.

2   **FOOD FIBER FUNDAMENTALS**

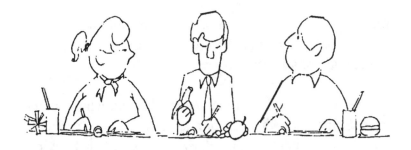

WHY ALL THE FUSS
THESE DAYS ABOUT FIBER?

F̲ew of us are aware how we spend our lives sandwiched between two populations of bacteria. We live between a modest collection of transient passengers on the skin, and a universe of easy riders in the colon. It's a jungle both places, but the one with the greatest day-to-day significance for us is not the one on the skin but the one within. There are more bacteria in the

17

normal colon than there are cells in the entire human body. And they live for the most part on the food we eat and what we can't digest: fiber.

The interactions of fiber and bacteria and other components of our diet are as complex and secret as the orchestrations of life in a pond. Working relationships have evolved over millions of years and we are still some distance from their full understanding. Digestion and nutrition and fiber are more complex than, say, the use of wheat bran for laxation or oat bran for a lower cholesterol.

Food fiber is found in fruits, vegetables and whole grains. By definition, it is that part of normal food which cannot be digested by normal processes in the normal human intestine. Some fibers look like textile fabric, some look flakey, while still others can be dissolved in water. What they all have in common is their indigestibility and their enormous size as molecules. Scaled up to human terms, if a food molecule such as sugar be imagined to be the size of a person, a fiber molecule would be 20 stories high and the length of several city blocks: a huge submarine sponge full of holes, tunnels, windows, halls and passageways.

This enormous size, relative to food molecules, is a major fiber property. Not only does it help them trap food particles but also to capture water for a laxative effect. These "capture properties" help distend the upper gut for appetite satisfaction, producing the sensation of fullness that assists with weight control. Lower down, trapped carcinogens are kept off the bowel wall and carried out of the body for an anti-cancer benefit.

By trapping food molecules, fiber keeps up to 10% of food calories out of reach of the digestive process, further helping with weight control. Lower in the gut, such particles are reduced by bacteria to hydrogen and carbon dioxide, gases that give the high fiber diet its reputation. Such flatulence is the sound of bacteria at work, serving their own interests while helping you control your weight. It should be music to the weight prone person's ears. Any change in the kind of food you eat leads to a change in the composition of the populations of bacteria in your digestive tract. There's extra turbulence, typically, during the early weeks with bubblings and gurglings that eventually settle down, although never to the lethal stillness of the low fiber state.

The silence of today's low fiber diet is the silence of disease at work. It is not a healthy stillness. An adequately fibered diet interacts with the digestive tract and with its denizens to produce a finely tuned instrument that can be expected to bubble merrily as a tea kettle, normally and healthily producing gas for release about once an hour.

"...AN INDUSTRIAL PROCESSING FATE WHOSE PREFERENCE HAS COST US MUCH FIBER AND NOT A LITTLE HEALTH. "

P erhaps nothing better illustrates the fate of fiber in today's diet than the orange. As a fruit for eating it has been swamped by the popularity of its juice. We've almost doubled orange consumption since 1970 to produce some 700 million gallons of juice a year; fresh, frozen, bottled or canned, an industrial processing fate whose preference has cost us all much fiber and not a little health.

Beyond the obvious effects on laxation and bowel health, some food fibers such as the pectin of oranges can capture cholesterol and help prevent heart attacks. Volunteers placed on low fat diets to reduce their cholesterol levels had starting levels of 220 that fell to 190; and when a pectin supplement was added to their program cholesterol levels fell further to 170. That's well below the normal upper limit of 200 recommended by the World Health Organization.

In a study of fiber and appetite satisfaction, 16 overweight college students were placed on 1,200 calorie-a-day weight control diets that included 12 slices of bread each day. The students were instructed to eat the bread and take as little or as much of the prescribed diet as they desired to control feelings of fatigue, headache or hunger. Half the students were given bright white bread. After two months, all the students had lost weight, but there was a difference. Those on white bread had lost an average of 14 pounds each, while those on high-fiber bread lost an average of 19 pounds each. That's a five pound improvement from the inclusion of a single fiber element.

One reason for the five pound difference in the study would be the result of fiber trapping calorie nutrients and preventing their absorption. This temporary trapping of nutrients high in the digestive tract and their subsequent release to bacterial action lower down, as well as their slower, almost metered delivery all along the gut, are now recognized contributions of fiber to greater appetite satisfaction, smoother absorption and easier weight control.

A pound of food, whether as steak or watermelon, fills most of us to satisfaction. A pound of food distends the stomach and signals the brain that enough is on board. The stomach is a staging area during digestion. It is a food blender of sorts whose job is to hold chunks of chewed and swallowed solid food until they are sufficiently liquefied for passage into the small intestine. Other signals, chemical in nature, are released from the stretched stomach walls and tell the appetite center in the brain that the drive to eat can be turned off. These crucial functions of the stomach in appetite satisfaction are bypassed by food refinement and fiber loss, by an orange defibered into orange juice.

From a practical standpoint, fiber in the diet comes from foods of vegetable origin. Fiber's role in the plant is to provide it with structure and protection. Given the wide variety in our intake of plant products, there are inevitably wide variations in the fiber intakes of individual Americans. The range is 20-60 grams per day or, in household terms, 4 to 12 teaspoons. Vegetarians generally eat the most, while heavy consumers of meat, chicken and fish usually eat the least. The best sources of fiber are fresh fruits and vegetables, peas, beans and lentils; as well as whole grain products.

" ...GASTRIC SURGERY IS AN ATTEMPT TO FORCE UPON THE MORBIDLY OBESE EATING HABITS THE RIGHT FOOD WOULD HELP PROVIDE."

As a society we are bigger than any before, even taller and more muscular than our relatives in Europe, Asia or Africa. And we are fatter. Between 1965 and 1985, already well-fed, we gained on average another eight pounds. In creating a culture of abundance, where consumption and ease is encouraged at every level, we have produced some conspicuous victims. They are the people in growing numbers whose body weights exceed the ideal by a hundred or more pounds and who can't stop the process. They are the morbidly obese and they are a challenge to the health care system.

Being morbidly obese is very bad news. It increases one's chance of disability or death twelvefold between the ages of 25 and 35, and sixfold between the ages of 35 and 45. When obese patients have stomach surgery for weight control, two chambers are created in the stomach - a tiny upper chamber connected through a small hole to a larger lower chamber. Food enters the upper chamber that has the capacity of only a couple of tablespoons so it fills quickly and begins to hurt. One particularly difficult patient of mine had his stomach reduced surgically. This meant that he would hurt whenever he ate more than a couple of tablespoons of food. He discovered he could defeat the surgery with ice cream, and he did.

Another surgical approach is gastric bypassing. This cuts the stomach off at the top and closes the bottom half. Then a loop of intestine is brought up from below and connected to the upper remnant of stomach. Still another procedure wraps the stomach tightly in a ribbon of plastic, reducing its total capacity to a two-ounce column. They're not for the faint-hearted, these interventions; they are desperate measures, indeed. Better to change one's ways.

In refining and processing food we have relieved it of much of its fiber and appetite satisfaction. Fiber in its way, does what surgical interventions attempt to do: slow the digestive process down. For anyone with a weight problem, begin slowing down your digestive process with whole food. New eating strategies ought to be built around whole grains, fruits and vegetables; foods that stay longer in the mouth and in the stomach. Gastric surgery is an attempt to force upon the morbidly obese eating habits that the right food itself would help provide.

A higher fiber diet would also help reduce cancer of the colon. Fiber helps capture the natural cancer causing agents that occur during digestion and sweeps them out of the system. Populations on high fiber diets have very little colon cancer. It's rare among Africans, yet black Americans have the same risk of colon cancer as white Americans. The disease is very rare in Africa because the diet is fiber laden. In any country that has no significant colon cancer problem, fiber intakes tend to be 3 times higher than ours. American vegetarians, black and white, also have a low risk of colon cancer. They consume about twice as much fiber as the average fellow citizen.

Beyond cancer protection, a 1984 study in Norway, demonstrated that fiber helped speed the healing of duodenal ulcers. It did this in competition with the milk and mush feeding traditionally prescribed. Fiber actually soothes and smooths. It's not roughage and toughage, but smoothage and soothage.

DISCOVER VEGETABLES
AND THEIR SEASONINGS

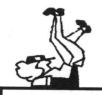 FITNESS FEEDINGS

TOASTED CARROTS

8 carrots, peeled and quartered lengthwise
plain yogurt
1 cup wheat germ

Steam or cook carrots until tender. Drain. Dip in plain yogurt and then roll in wheat germ. Place on a baking sheet sprayed with Pam. Bake at 350 degrees for 15 minutes or until toasted. Each serving equals two carrots.

CARROTS AND SCALLIONS

2-21/2 cups steamed carrots, sliced or julienned
1 tsp. Ginger-Garlic Oil
2-3 chopped scallions (green part only)

Briefly saute scallions in oil. Add the carrots and heat through.

COACH'S CORNER

LOOKING GOOD / FEELING BETTER

The things we're eating these days are not making us what we want to be. Accumulating evidence shows them to be tightly associated with heart disease, cancer and obesity.

Excessive salt intakes are related to high blood pressure, while excessive food refinement promotes obesity, diabetes, diverticulitis and bowel cancer. The best-tasting, most convenient, affordable and abundant food in the world carries a health cost.

So people in growing numbers are beginning to change their food intakes in the interest of feeling better and looking better. They're returning to an older, less glittering more peaceful foodstyle, one on which humankind evolved and one to which the human digestive tract accomodates quickly and quietly, and gratefully.

It's a health-promoting, reassuring foodstyle, and its preparation calls for a minimum of fuss and stress. It's mainstays are uncomplicated dishes, vegetable soups, pastas, breads and salads. Its foods are quick to fix and rely on such convenience techology as the freezer, the blender and the microwave oven. There's still a lot of nutritious, delicious user-friendly food in your local supermarket.

27

LAXATION FUNDAMENTALS

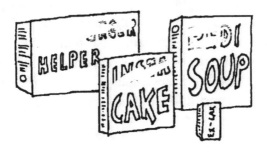

HOW ARE LAXATION AND HEALTH RELATED?

In lots of ways, but let's start with constipation if only because doctors and patients usually disagree on their definitions of it. More than 10,000 adults were interviewed as part of a major national survey in 1985 and 70% reported a daily bowel movement. Whether the remaining 30 % suffer from constipation is at issue.

The interviewers in the study defined constipation in terms of laxative use, but the consistency of the bowel movement is the best indication of the state of laxation ... too hard and you have constipation (regardless of frequency), too soft (or liquid) and you have diarrhea.

29

Water makes up 90% of stool weight. Without water, food residue, also known as fiber, normally makes up a third of the dry weight of each bowel movement. Food residue enters the large bowel from the small bowel carried by 20 quarts of digestive juice each 24 hour day. Along with the fiber, sheets of cells that line the gut are normally shed into the stool each day. They enter the large bowel to provide about another third of the dry weight of stool. Finally, in the large bowel are enormous numbers of proliferating bacteria that constitute the final third of the dry weight of stool.

The most important job of the large bowel is to recover those 20 quarts of digestive fluid for recycling back into the body. Food fiber competes with this recovery function by holding fluid in the residue and bulking the stool up. A high-fiber diet is a stool-softening diet because water is held against the extraction forces of the large bowel.

The longer the time that residue stays in the large bowel the more prolonged the opportunity for bowel muscle and lining cells to continue fluid extraction, and the harder and dryer the resulting residue. The shorter the time, the softer the residue. About 18 hours is the usual transit time that food residue takes to travel along the large bowel.

Researchers into constipation have found that a low-fiber intake is not as compromising of normal function as are other variables: age, inactivity, and food sensitivity.

Twice as many people in their early seventies (35%) had difficulty moving their bowels as among those under 30 (15%). Among men at every age level, those with low physical activity reported 15 times the rate of constipation as those who were physically active. Constipation was three times greater among sedentary women as among physically active women. It probably has to do with a jostling effect on the colon that speeds transit times.

> ## "PRODUCING CARCINOGENS IS A NORMAL RESULT OF DIGESTION ... THEY ARE DILUTED AND MADE LESS TOXIC BY THE WATER HELD BY FIBER."

The job of the large bowel, as a drying and storage section of the digestive tract, is to recover the 20 quarts of fluid delivered into it every day. Food nutrients are not absorbed from it, once the products of digestion arrive there. Its principle activities are compacting, storage and discharge. Approximately 4 times a day, major isolated segments of the large bowel contract in a slow, compressing action that expresses from bowel content water and gases to be absorbed back into the circulation. At other times, and throughout the day, less dramatic and gentler kneading actions take place along its entire length for similar drying and compacting purposes. Fiber helps in this process by holding water in the bowel and preventing excessive drying of its contents. This eases laxation and keeps the pressures low. It also reduces the risk of producing tiny balloons of diverticulitis from excessive pressures.

A diverticulum is a small outpouching or ballooning of bowel, usually not even as large as the tip of one's little finger. It forms at points of weakness in the bowel, typically where blood vessels enter an opening in the muscle of the bowel wall. If they become painfully inflamed the condition is called diverticulitis. It's a common condition among adult Americans that increases with age, and is practically unknown in populations on high-fiber diets; observations that gave impetus to the monkey research outlined next.

The monkeys clearly didn't like the study, but the researchers who inserted pressure recording balloons into their colons found answers to many questions regarding diverticulitis. Studies on the monkeys demonstrated that low fiber diets such as the average American eats, allow high pressure to be generated by these contractions inside the bowel, thus ballooning out any weaknesses along the bowel wall. In the monkey study, pressures went 3 times as high as the pressures generated on a well-fibered diet.

So the research tells us that an early element in the production of diverticulitis is a lifelong low-fiber diet resulting in large bowel pressures which eventually find weak points to bubble. Fiber keeps bowel pressures down by trapping water, maintaining bulk and preventing bowel muscle from exerting its full force to cause diverticulitis. A bulky stool also speeds transit time, easing laxation.

The longer that food residues stay in the large bowel, the greater the opportunity for mischief. The longer that colon bacteria act upon and react with incompletely digested food products, the greater the potential for a build-up of carcinogens. Producing carcinogens is a normal result of digestion. They are generated every day in the large bowel from the interaction of food, bile and bacteria. They are diluted and made less toxic by the water held by fiber. It is a process whose potentially bad effects are minimized by daily evacuation and by dilution with fiber-held water.

Finally, for certain susceptible individuals, common foods can be constipating, or "binding" as they are often described. It's a common phenomenon called food sensitivity resulting in recurring episodes of sinus congestion, headache, day-long muscle or joint aches, fatigue, bloating, weight swings, and constipation characterized by pellet-like stools. The symptoms are produced by food such as wheat products, or corn, or chocolate, etc. Symptoms tend to take a day or two to show themselves after the food has been eaten so the relationship may not be recognized. See the discussion of this common and commonly unrecognized problem in Part II.

33

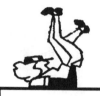

FITNESS FEEDINGS

CLEAN BLACK BEAN SOUP

1 cup black beans
4 cups water
Boil beans in water for 2 minutes; cover, let sit 2 hours, drain and discard water.

1/2 tsp oregano
1/2 tsp thyme
2 T wine vinegar
1/2 tsp hot pepper sauce
1 T sherry
1 tsp sugar - optional
3-1/2 cups Chicken Stock
2/3 cup chopped onion
1/2 cup chopped green pepper
1 clove garlic, mashed
1 bay leaf
Combine cooked, drained beans, stock, onion, garlic, green pepper, oregano, thyme, vinegar, and bay leaf. Bring to a boil, cover and simmer at least 1 hour or until beans are tender. Add pepper and cook 5 minutes more. Adjust seasonings. Remove bay leaf. Puree half of the beans and return to the soup. Freezes beautifully.

COACH'S CORNER

TIPS ON CHANGING HABITS

1) Take inventory of your starting assets. Don't overlook what you've got. Then set small reasonable goals and work toward them from where you are.

2) Start with whatever is easiest or most agreeable and has the quickest return on your effort. Overcome inertia.

3) Don't rush to get it all completed by tomorrow. Life is a process, a process of change and becoming.

4) Learn to do as much as you can without outside help or involvement. Do it for yourself.

5) Let family, friends and even strangers enrich your life but not burden it. Let them in on your plans and projects. Share a few secrets.

AEROBIC FITNESS FUNDAMENTALS

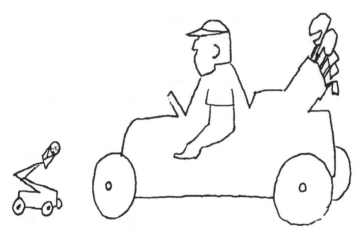

IS FITNESS ALL ITS CRACKED UP TO BE?

T he hopes that most of us have for a long and healthy life are dashed by the development of a fatal disease like cancer or symptomatic coronary artery disease in our middle years. Compared to inactive people, however, active individuals get less cancer and have fewer heart attacks, and if they do get hit by either, it's much later in life.

37

Studies on more than 5,000 female alumni who graduated between 1924 and 1981 from ten Boston area colleges indicated that the regular exercisers got less female cancer. The data allowed for such modifying factors as age, cancer family history, pregnancies, estrogens, obesity and smoking. Correcting for all those variables, fitness was still associated with a reduced risk of breast and reproduction system cancer.

Also from Boston comes another fitness study on more than 20,000 male Harvard alumni and it focused on heart attacks. Continuing fitness benefits were easily demonstrated, and found to be "dose" responsive. The more exercise they got each week, the proportionately lower the risk of heart attack.

From a biological perspective, the proportionality of benefits to effort is important: It signifies a dose-response relationship. Had the better health observed among the fit been a result of other unrecognized characteristics, no proportional relationship would have resulted. Their genes would have conferred equal protection. Individuals who covered 20 miles a week on foot had fewer heart deaths than individuals who covered 10 miles a week on foot, who in turn had fewer heart attacks than those who covered fewer or none. The Harvard finding also demonstrated that the benefits were not storable. Being fit as an undergraduate did not lead to heart protection in later years unless the fitness was maintained. By the same token, sedentary and non-athletic undergraduates who took up fitness later in life were found to receive heart protective benefits.

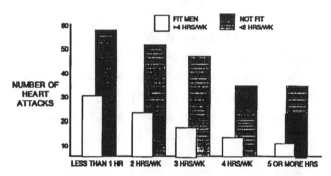

EFFECTS OF FITNESS ON HEART ATTACKS
THE LONG TERM HARVARD ALUMNI STUDY

REGARDLESS OF UNDERGRADUATE HABITS, LIFELONG HABITS COUNT THE MOST

Whether they were Harvard graduates or not, within days of being immobilized with broken backs, healthy young men begin a decline in brain function. As each week progresses their ability to memorize a random set of numbers declines. Then it gradually begins a return to pre-fracture levels with healing and ambulation.

Beyond helping postpone premature death from heart disease and cancer, fitness also benefits the brain and mood by putting quality into the additional years. It generates energy and improves performance. The energy generated increases confidence, self-esteem, and supports a feeling of optimism. All these benefits slow both the physiological and social withdrawal of aging.

One neurological sign of aging, for example, is the speed at which nerve pulses are transmitted. In the older individual, slower transmission speeds and reaction times are the rule, and these too, improve with physical activity . Men in their 70's who have been fit for a decade have reaction times that are faster than those of sedentary men half their age.

In the state of Utah, fitness was found to benefit a population of retirees across the board. They were divided into three groups: sedentary, stretch and tone, and walking. Within three months there was an improvement in mood and memory in the second two groups but mostly in the group that walked. In studies on middle-aged rats, exercised rats not only developed brains that performed better, but brains that actually enlarged as a result of the exercise. The probable mechanism of the enlargement is epinephrine. During exercise its levels increase in the blood that bathes the brain. Studies of brain tissue in an incubator dish have shown that epinephrine promotes brain cell proliferation or growth.

Bone and joint fitness benefits have been well documented. Turkey wing studies demonstrate that exercise holds calcium in the bones. The astronauts in space lose calcium from their bones unless they do calisthenics, and studies on lifelong runners in Florida indicate that 10, 15 or 20 years of running for an average of 30 miles a week has no bad effect on normal knees. Joints are nourished by physical activity, not worn down. The mechanism of this benefit is the compressible surface cartilage acts like a squeegee to absorb and retain joint fluid.

"... IT INVOLVES GETTING TO KNOW THE ANIMAL WITHIN, ITS CARE AND FEEDING."

A fit adult individual is one who can cover 5 miles on foot within an hour without suffering undue strain on the breathing and cardiovascular system nor undue consequences after. A fit individual has a resting heart rate of 60 beats per minute and a resting blood pressure of 110/70. Fitness comes from easy uninterrupted effort over time.

T he bipedal facts of life indicate that we did not evolve as sedentary creatures; that we are muscled to rely on our hind legs and a wide variety of balancing muscles to move in the upright position; and that the greatest return on effort comes from exercises undertaken on our two feet...walking, dancing, jogging, running, skipping rope, rebounding, etc. Pedestrian activities such as golf or bowling (or even tennis for the most part) do not provide aerobic benefits because they are interrupted. Machines or equipment that enable you to sit down or to float or to lie back do not provide the benefit of comparable effort on foot. Physical activity also benefits the brain, whether you're a Harvard graduate or not.

Chemicals are turned loose in the body during activity that have a stimulating effect on the brain. The best documented ones are the hormones adrenalin and (its cousin) noradrenalin. The more sustained the effort, the higher and more prolonged their resulting elevations and benefits. They are get-up-and-go hormones, the survival signals to all tissues of the body for fight or flight. They stimulate and probably make us smarter. Noting that the brain of the domestic rabbit was smaller than the brain of the wild rabbit, Darwin speculated that perhaps it reflected a lack of stimulation. The wild rabbit is smarter than the domestic rabbit.

During a period of exercise, adrenalin soaks all tissues of the body including the brain. It speeds up all processes. It

42

would provoke sensations of panic or fear released at rest, but during exercise, and for several hours thereafter, it produces a feeling of increased energy, alertness, and the reassurance of readiness for performance. It is a confidence-building state of affairs. The hesitation and delays that are characteristic of age are rolled back. Compared to controls, the fitness group in Utah improved their memories, their ability to solve problems, their moods and their sleep-waking patterns. Both groups started the same. Fitness consisted of covering three miles a day on foot within an hour, and its benefits were measurable within six weeks.

"TO GET YOUR WEIGHT UNDER CONTROL YOU GET FIT, AND TO GET YOUR HEART UNDER CONTROL YOU DIET. REALLY. "

Finally, there's the national weight problem. Weight loss without exercise burns calories from the body's muscle tissue as well as its fat stores. A weight loss of 30 pounds that is half muscle and half fat reduces the muscle mass of the body by about 15 pounds. It is usually a permanent muscle loss for inactive people, a loss of metabolically busy tissue that leads to a reduced need for calories down the road. Even at rest, muscle tissue burns calories faster

43

than fat tissue. Losing muscle tissue during the calorie restriction of a weight loss diet is a long-term disaster for weight control.

In a recent weight loss study, a group of overweight volunteers were placed on restricted diets of 1,000 calories a day. Half of them were also put on a walking program for 30 minutes each day, while the other half were not. After two months on the program, the "diet only" half had lost 20 pounds while the "diet walking" half had lost 23 pounds. Not a very impressive added benefit from the walking--three pounds over two months--but the difference in body composition was remarkable and foretold a very different future for the two groups.

All subjects had been measured at the start and finish for their total body fat and total muscle by underwater weighing. The walking group had gained two pounds of muscle which masked their total loss of 25 pounds of fat. The non-walking group had lost 8 pounds of muscle and 12 pounds of fat. On the surface they had roughly the same weight change but very different sub-surface outcomes: 25 pounds of fat lost by the walkers compared to 12 by the diet onlies. And their future energy requirements will be different too. The diet-only group will gain weight much more easily thanks to their smaller muscle mass.

So common is this experience, that the average patient in her middle years who has crash dieted several times to lose the same 20 or 30 pounds has progressively reduced her body's muscle mass in exchange for fat. Then she adds only fat with each regain. This so lowers the metabolically active tissue in her body that she routinely gains weight on the standard 1200 calorie diet prescribed by her physician.

Repeated episodes of weight loss from crash dieting have a lasting impact on body composition. With each loss/regain cycle there's less lean muscle tissue and more fat tissue at the same weight on the bathroom scale. With each complete swing cycle, body fat slowly climbs from 30% to 40% to 50% of total body weight, and because fat is bulkier (ounce-for-ounce) than muscle, clothing sizes keep climbing at the same scale weight. The progress can only be checked by using one's muscles during periods of weight loss, by walking for example.

There's no alternative for the overweight individual. No free lunch. Regular daily walks are essential. Otherwise, with each crash program cycle, muscle is slowly exchanged for fat and the furnace flame becomes a pilot light.

In summary, the two greatest errors that the average individual makes with regard to weight and heart attacks are that to get your weight under control, you diet, and to get your heart under control you get fit. Surprise! It's the other way around. Really. For weight control, fitness is the most important element in your lifestyle. For heart attack prevention, diet change gets highest priority.

FITNESS FEEDINGS

APPLE-OATMEAL MUFFINS

3/4 cup rolled oats
1 cup whole wheat flour
3 tsp baking powder
1 tsp cinnamon
1 cup skim milk
2 egg whites, slightly beaten
2 T molasses
1 cup grated apple, peeled or unpeeled
2 T oil

Combine dry ingredients. Add oil, egg, milk and molasses. Mix well. Add apple and mix. Spoon into greased muffin pan. Bake 20 minutes in a preheated 400 degree oven. Makes 12-16 muffins.

COACH'S CORNER

THE BEST FITNESS ACTIVITIES

WALKING: Human beings have been walking upright for over a million years. It is a simple activity, once the basics are mastered, and requires no special equipment or training. It is safe and available year round. It tones up most of the body's muscles as well as the heart and lungs. It is a natural tranquilizer. It can be very sociable. For anyone beginning a fitness program, walking is the basic unit of effort. Start out with it.

DANCING: For many people dancing is a pleasant alternative to walking or jogging. And they are right. Many women, exhausted by even the prospect of a 10 minute walk can dance for hours, given agreeable music and company. Dancing is an excellent combination of a fitness activity and recreation. So are skating, skipping rope and rebounding.

JOGGING: There is no shortage of horror stories for anyone thinking about starting to run: the overweight fellow who starts to jog and is found dead along the road or the middle-age heart attack victim who quits smoking, loses weight, starts to exercise and has his second heart attack. Jogging is graduate level walking. Don't start with it, and when you do, start slowly.

5 RECREATION FUNDAMENTALS

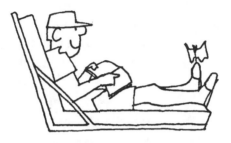

JUST WHAT IS RE-CREATION IN TISSUE TERMS?

O ne essential to full health and peak performance is an escape hatch from pressures. You need a strategy that gets you unwound, or provides a mental break when you can't leave your desk. Hobbies, books and the arts provide traditional re-creation opportunities off the job, but for immediate help, some kind of controlled relaxation is a good escape hatch. There's nothing mysterious about it. All you need is a quiet place or a mental device (like a soft word you repeat to yourself in a rhythmic and hypnotic way such as the word "one, one, one'). You are trying to produce a relaxed body.

49

Back off for a moment and regard the situation that lead up to the need for a break. During the day's obligations you are engaged in a state of concentration. Your mental energy tends to be concentrated on pre-occupying concerns. Tension builds in body muscles and fatigue sets in, events that can occur over an hour or so, a day or two or a week or more. Repair and recharging are required, and time must be taken.

For really short breaks remove all signs of time - close your eyes for a bit, or you take off your watch and put it in a drawer. Release your attention to your own internal rhythms and not the ticking clock. Set an alarm if you can. If possible put your feet up, shoes off, clothes loose, lights down, surroundings warm and quiet. Let it all go for the short break. You are scratching and satisfying a secret itch. And it feels good. Recreation re-creates.

Another escape involves laughter. When writer-editor Norman Cousins ascribed his escape from debilitating disease to laughter, he meant it. Hours of funny films, from Chaplin to the Three Stooges over several weeks had him in stitches and out of his sick bed. A good belly laugh is a form of release, a burst of internal, visceral energy. Anyone who has fallen out of a chair laughing, has demonstrated its loosening effect .

Finding time for humor or play means imposing order on

your day. Most of us pack as much as we can into any given day, and we overload it. We get much done but never everything, so we feel pressured by time and deadlines, playing the game of beat the clock and not the game of wellness. Learn to delegate. Follow reasonable time tables. Minimize time spent spinning wheels. And make space in each day to slip your engine into idle for a few minutes.

Wellness is a process that requires daily balancing. Your needs, wants and obligations must be regularly re-alligned. Studies have shown that we function best on a 12-hour cycle, starting at 6 in the morning and ending at 6 in the evening. Each day is most in sync with our tissues if it follows the rhythm of the sun, the time giver of most of the body's clocks. When ignored, it creates dysrhythms that reflect themselves in bad feelings and poor performance.

Those paragons of the work ethic the bee, the ant and the beaver only work about a third of the day. A third of the time they rest, and a third of the time they just seem to be knocking about the neighborhood. Do likewise.

FITNESS FEEDINGS

STIR-FRY PROCEDURE FOR ONE-DISH MEALS

Starting the night before or that morning, have 2-3 cups of vegetables (any three or more) cleaned and trimmed to size, preferably thinly sliced. Almost any vegetables will do.

At cooking time, heat 1-2 tsp of Ginger-Garlic Seasoned Oil and 2-3 T Chicken Stock and 1-2 T sherry in a wok or skillet. Use the highest setting. Add the vegetables and toss and stir until tender/crisp - don't overcook.

Remove with a slotted spoon. To the liquid in the pan, add: 1 T cornstarch dissolved in 1/3 cup cool water or chicken stock. Cook over low heat, stirring until slightly thickened. Sparingly add tamari to taste. Return vegetables to the wok or skillet and heat through.

Serve over your choice of grain or beans. This is especially good over barley, bulgur or brown rice.

COACH'S CORNER

SOME RE-CREATING OPTIONS

1) Do something frivolous or unexpected - give a gift for no reason, take the week-end off at a local motel.

2) Cook up a special dish or drive 100 miles to a really great restaurant or great shopping mall.

3) Activate an old or develop a new hobby. Work on needlepoint, a jigsaw puzzle, or sort photos. Get a computer and learn some new games.

4) Send out some job resumes. You might be pleasantly surprised at what you stir up.

5) Spend an hour in a book store or your library. You'll be amazed at what you fancy.

6) Go somewhere with an unlimited view - the beach, the mountains, the desert. Find some wild water that's crashing around and listen to it for a while.

7) Join a group that does politics, plays the market or helps others.

PART TWO

MAJOR LEAGUE HEALTH ISSUES

1 AN OVERVIEW OF FUNDAMENTALS

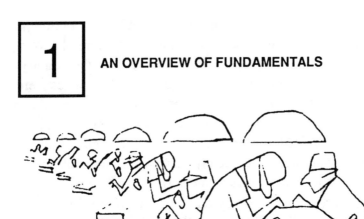

HIGH TECH AND HIGH HOPES

A national study involving thousands of participants over a 10 year period, was completed in the mid 1980s and demonstrated that lowering blood cholesterol levels does help prevent heart attacks. It was one of many studies over the past two decades but it was the most significant because it began an education campaign for the general public and the nation's doctors that's now up to speed in the 1990s.

It's not going to be an easy job, however, and for reasons that have little to do with public acceptance of a new foodstyle. One problem concerns the nation's laboratories. They tend to mislead regarding normal cholesterol levels. In a 1988 survey of 100 laboratories around the country, researchers concluded that the laboratories themselves were a major reason that only 10% of physicians were taking action to lower their patients' cholesterol levels. Blood measures are accurate enough but their high upper range of normal values lulls too many participants into inactivity. Cholesterol experts agree that normal adult levels should not exceed 200 but many cite data supporting 180 as the upper normal limit. Too many of the nation's laboratories accompany their measurements with reassurances that questionable levels are normal.

"...THE SECOND MOST COMMON BLOOD VESSEL OPERATION WORLDWIDE."

Another problem for cholesterol educators is the quick fix preference of surgery for the cholesterol problem. Most surgical procedures involve veins taken from the leg and used to bypass narrowed arteries on the surface of the heart. The procedure was pioneered in the 1960s in Argentina, refined in Canada and accepted as a treatment of choice in the U.S. It's now a $10 billion annual industry whose less-than-satisfactory results have led to competing alternatives: Implants of chest wall arteries into narrowed heart arteries, or selective balloon expansion of the tunnel of a narrowed artery. The first-mentioned alternate permanently borrows blood from the chest wall by re-directing it into heart muscle. The second involves inserting a deflated balloon, positioning it over the soft cholesterol deposits and squashing them flat by inflating the balloon. It takes advantage of the patchy distribution of cholesterol pimples, flattening the mountains by filling in the valleys.

A follow-up report from Switzerland where the balloon procedure was pioneered, reveals that among the first 169 patients in whom ballooning was performed, closure occurred during the first six months in 30% of the patients and in another 30% over the next two years. It buys some time, perhaps several years.

A variety of new techniques are under study which involve vaporizing cholesterol deposits with laser beam technology, reaming them out with tiny augers, or inserting small tubes called stents. All of these efforts are interesting and worthy, and under study in centers around the world, but they are very early in their development. The lining of the artery is a fragile thing. It must be kept intact or it will encourage blood to clot. Funneling, tunneling and burning techniques have two major shortcomings: They damage the delicate lining that the cholesterol deposits lie under, and they are focal in their approach. The disease involves all arteries of the heart and body throughout their lengths, and mechanical interventions cannot reach 90% of the system.

One new technique, however, that is quite promising is blood scrubbing. In this process blood is removed from the patient (as with a blood bank donation) cycled through a scrubbing apparatus which selectively removes cholesterol then returns the clean blood to the patient. It takes about four hours to lower cholesterols from a very high to a very low. To assess its benefits, patients taking part in this approach are having angiograms (artery pictures) done of their coronaries every month. Early reports indicate that the procedure produces generalized regression, and if promise holds, this would appear to be the technology of the future... simple, ambulatory, and an intervention that goes with the grain of the process rather than across it.

For the rest of this decade, however, knowing your cholesterol level, getting it down under 180 and keeping it there is the essence of effectively preventing heart attacks.

"...THE PROSPECT OF CUTTING ONE'S FAT
INTAKE IN HALF PRODUCES A FLAVOR
CRISIS IN MOST MOUTHS."

N ot only the heart, but all the body's structures require an adequate blood supply. Cholesterol deposits in the heart are associated with deposits everywhere in the body. Noises from deposits in the large arteries of the neck can begin to be heard with the examining stethoscope in about 5% of individuals over the age of 45. The incidence increases to 25% by age 70. The noises come from turbulence in the bloodstream as it travels over the accumulating lumps in the walls of the arteries. Like the sounds of rapids, they are strong indications of turbulence in the system from narrowing projections into the artery tunnel.

They are often eventually associated with a stroke, so a surgical procedure was developed and used in hope of preventing that outcome. Called carotid endarterectomy, candidates for the procedure usually are discovered to have noisy neck arteries and may report transient episodes of one-sided weakness. During this procedure, the surgeon removes accumulations of cholesterol from the large arteries in the neck, the carotid arteries that serve the brain. Next to coronary artery bypass surgery this procedure is the second most common blood vessel operation worldwide. Nearly 100,000 U.S. patients undergo it every year, yet only recently have the hoped-for benefits been properly evaluated.

In one study reported from Toronto, 500 patients considered to be ideal candidates for the treatment were randomly assigned to have the operation or not have it. All were managed as well as possible with medication.

The Toronto researchers reported no benefit from the surgery in preventing strokes compared to non-surgical management. During the year of follow-up, 5 patients in each group of 250 subsequently suffered a stroke. Of interest additionally, and highlighting the generalized nature of this disorder, was that more patients in both populations suffered heart attacks than strokes, 8 compared to 5. And their heart attacks were more often fatal than heart attacks in the general population. Cholesterol deposits produce disease in all arteries of the body, most dramatically in the heart and brain.

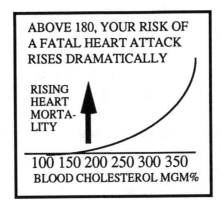

So neck artery surgery doesn't reduce the risk of stroke, and mortality from the procedure itself runs about 3%. It's a procedure that has been measured and found wanting. Concluded other researchers reporting on other ineffective surgical interventions for narrowed brain arteries: "Alas, the negative results of this study no longer allow us to believe that surgery is a instrument of consequence in the prevention of stroke."

C holesterol disease, whatever blood vessels it involves clinically, is at root a nutrition and metabolic disease, best managed by lowering blood cholesterol levels to begin the process of healing through disease regression. Given half a chance, arteries are self-cleaning. But the prospect of cutting one's fat intake in half produces a flavor crisis in most mouths. It is a radical food change because the percentage of calories in our diet from fat over this century has gone up steadily, from 30% to 40%. That's not a 10% increase but a 30% increase, historically huge. Since 1980, during one decade alone, the national consumption of edible oils has gone from 45 to 58 pounds a year. It's an oil slick health ride that coincides with the national weight and heart problem. Reducing the fats and oils begins the process of risk factor control, of which the research tells us there are many. What about a little help in all this from science? Would any supplements help here?

Well, there's a pharmaceutical fiber called cholestyramine which Boston researchers have found to be effective. They were as interested in its cost as in its clinical effectiveness, however, and their study involved men 35 to 75 with elevated levels of blood cholesterol followed for 5 years. The annual cost of treatment was $700 per person per year, which works out to about $36,000 of medication per year of life saved.

Even the researchers thought it looked like a lot to be

64

paying for benefits that could be achieved in a less costly way, as Italian researchers have already discovered. Replacing animal protein with plant protein was their less expensive way to reduce blood cholesterol. After 16 weeks, 19 patients given bean protein instead of animal protein had a 30% reduction in blood cholesterol levels. In other subjects given plant-protein supplements such as soy protein drinks, cholesterol levels were reduced by 30%. Plant proteins, as replacements for meat or as dietary supplements have a cost effective role to play for individuals and organizations concerned about medical costs.

Between these technical extremes, the bypassing or scrubbing, and the soybean extracts, there's a laxative supplement that also lowers cholesterol. It's called psyllium and its correct name is psyllium hydrophilic muciloid. Taking one or two teaspoons three times a day has lowered cholesterol levels by 15% in a group of 13 men after only two months, without any change in their diets. Taking that kind of supplement at a rate of 20 cents a day compares well to soy or cholestyramine. And think how they'd benefit from an assist in the better food habits department.

Supplements or not, surgery or not, everything intended to improve heart health begins with a diet low in fat and cholesterol, and high in fiber. And for most individuals, truth to tell, these may be the only changes necessary.

MEET ANOTHER SCORE CARD

On the opposite page you'll find five categories of food and other habits that contribute in major ways to today's health concerns.

FATS AND OILS AND CHOLESTEROL HABITS: Lead to weight problems, cancer and to heart attacks. Not only are fats and oils identified, but cholesterol sources as well.

FOOD SALT SOURCES: Makes food tasty but can raise the blood pressure of susceptible individuals. There are many more sources of salt in today's diet than those identified so enter your favorite if it's not listed.

BIOSTRESS ISSUES: Feelings of anxiety or anger are common. They are action moods for which physical action is rarely taken in our culture. The result is unreleased tension. See Stress Fundamentals, Chapter 5.

LIFESTYLE ISSUES: Activities grouped here are common, everyday practices for managing pain. While they do provide temporary relief from stress, they are also indicators of health problems in one's life.

FOOD INDUCED ACHES AND PAINS. Many people experience chronic nasal congestion, chronic headache or chronic abdominal symptoms that are all food-related. They are not life-threatening, but they are certainly life-disrupting. A good approach is to avoid those foods responsible. See Sensitivity Fundamentals, Chapter 7.

As for how my obliging patient, Martin K, did with this one, please turn the page.

2. READING ALL THE PITCHES

(NOTE THE NEW AND _REVERSED_ SCORING)

SCORING: DAILY: 0   WEEKLY: 5   MONTHLY: 10
(MORE OR LESS)   (TWICE OR THRICE)   (SELDOM OR NEVER)

		SCORING	
		You	**Ideal**
FOOD FATS & OILS & CHOLESTEROL*			
	BURGERS* / BACON-HAM* / FRANKS* / COLD CUTS*:		10
	% MILKS* / ICE CREAM* / CHEESE* / BUTTER*:		10
	DRESSINGS °/ MARG/MAYO* / FRIES° / PIZZA*/ RIBS*°:		10
GREASEBALL	CHIPS° / SNAX°/ SWEET ROLLS° / CAKE-PIE-COOKIES:°□		5
	BEEF-PORK-CHICKEN-TURKEY-FISH-SHRIMP*/ YOLK*:		5
FOOD SALT SOURCES			
	CANNED SOUPS/ COLD CEREALS/ PICKLES/ CHEESE:		5
SALTY SLIDER	PKGED. DINNERS, DESSERTS, SNACKS*/ EATING OUT:°□ ... °□		5
BIOSTRESS ISSUES			
	ANGRY : IRRITABLE-AGGRAVATED-TENSE:		5
	ANXIOUS : PRESSURED-DEADLINED-TENSE:		5
	BURNEDOUT: BORED-DISINTERESTED-DEPRESSED:		10
LIFESTYLE ISSUES			
	SICK DAYS-DRUGS-TABLETS-PILLS-ASPIRIN:		10
BEANBALL	LIQUOR-BEER-WINE-SMOKING / OTHER CHEMICALS:		10
FOOD-INDUCED ACHES , PAINS & CONGESTIONS			
	HEAD : HEADACHES / SINUS /NASAL STUFFINESS:		10
	CHEST : TIGHTNESS / PHLEGM / WHEEZING-COUGH:		10
SCREWBALL	ABDOMEN : ACHES / TENDERNESS / GAS / BLOATING:		10

*
- · HIGH IN CHOLESTEROL
- □ MAY CONTAIN CHOLESTEROL (BUTTER, EGG YOLK)
- ° MAY RAISE CHOLESTEROL (SAT. FATS, TRANS FATS)

YOUR PITCHES SCORE:	120
BASE RUNNING SCORE:	120
TOTAL PERFORMANCE	240

MARTIN K READS THE PITCHES

Martin approached this scorecard with trepidation. He appreciated the health significance of the categories and he didn't have to keep reminding himself that zeros, or daily frequencies, were bad news; he was already aware that the All American Diet was cholesterol laden, so he was not surprised to score low in the FOOD FATS AND OILS AND CHOLESTEROL.

A pamphlet distributed at his office concerning SALT AND HEALTH had alerted him to the effect of salt on his blood pressure level and to the fact that much of today's food is salt laden. He decided to think about it later.

BIOSTRESS ISSUES puzzled him. He was an even tempered man for the most part, happily married with two children. He decided that such anger as he did experience in the course of a week was work related and could more properly be called impatience, so he scored himself generously in this category.

He admitted much later to me that when he reached the LIFESTYLE ISSUES category he felt a twinge of guilt. He had been thinking of doing something about the daily booze "one-of-these-days" and apparently that time had come. He decided to reduce his consumption sharply.

With FOOD INDUCED ACHES, PAINS AND CONGESTIONS, he decided it didn't apply to him and he was correct in that assumption.

Finally, he added up his scores, the Base Running and Reading Pitches, for a rating on his Total Performance. The lowly total bothered him, always an achiever.

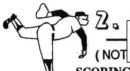

MARTIN K

(NOT ~~~~ G)

SCORING: DAILY: 0   **WEEKLY: 5**   **MONTHLY: 10**
(MORE OR LESS)   (TWICE OR THRICE)   (SELDOM OR NEVER)

SCORING

	FOOD FATS & OILS & CHOLESTEROL*	You	Ideal
	BURGERS* / BACON-HAM* / FRANKS* / COLD CUTS*:	0	10
	% MILKS* / ICE CREAM* / CHEESE* / BUTTER*:	0	10
	DRESSINGS / MARG/MAYO* / FRIES° / PIZZA*/ RIBS*:	5	10
	CHIPS / SNAX/ SWEET ROLLS / CAKE-PIE-COOKIES:	5	5
GREASEBALL	BEEF-PORK-CHICKEN-TURKEY-FISH-SHRIMP*/ YOLK*	0	5
	FOOD SALT SOURCES		
	CANNED SOUPS/ COLD CEREALS/ PICKLES/ CHEESE:	0	5
SALTY SLIDER	PKGED. DINNERS, DESSERTS, SNACKS*/ EATING OUT:	5	5
	BIOSTRESS ISSUES		
	ANGRY : IRRITABLE-AGGRAVATED-TENSE:	5	5
	ANXIOUS : PRESSURED-DEADLINED-TENSE:	10	5
	BURNEDOUT: BORED-DISINTERESTED-DEPRESSED:	10	10
	LIFESTYLE ISSUES		
BEANBALL	SICK DAYS-DRUGS-TABLETS-PILLS-ASPIRIN:	10	10
	LIQUOR-BEER-WINE-SMOKING / OTHER CHEMICALS:	0	10
	FOOD-INDUCED ACHES, PAINS & CONGESTIONS		
	HEAD : HEADACHES / SINUS /NASAL STUFFINESS:	10	10
	CHEST : TIGHTNESS / PHLEGM / WHEEZING-COUGH:	10	10
SCREWBALL	ABDOMEN : ACHES / TENDERNESS / GAS / BLOATING:	10	10

oh' oh

not me

*
- HIGH IN CHOLESTEROL
- ☐ MAY CONTAIN CHOLESTEROL (BUTTER, EGG YOLK)
- ° MAY RAISE CHOLESTEROL (SAT. FATS, TRANS FATS)

YOUR PITCHES SCORE: 80 | 120

BASE RUNNING SCORE: 40 | 120

TOTAL PERFORMANCE 120 | 240

MARTIN K'S NEXT REACTION

Once again, reinforced discouragement best described his mood, along with some tiny bat squeaks of alarm.

Time to straighten out some kinks in my lifestyle, he said to himself, and was reminded of Mark Twain's comment about changing bad habits ... "not by throwing them out the window, but by dragging them down the stairs one step at a time."

COACH'S CORNER

ON A CLEAR DAY

If we could see the condition of our arteries as readily as we see our complexions, most of us would have begun to change our ways years ago. The arteries of the average American begin to develop pimples of cholesterol during teenage years. Here and there they occur, slowly over the months and years, bumps of waxy cholesterol that collect to produce a kind of acne in the arteries, discoloring and disfiguring blemishes over a surface that should normally be as pale and slick as wet ice.

It's all out of sight of course, and unlike ordinary acne, artery acne does not usually heal or disappear. It grows over the years until it projects into the center of the artery, closing it off suddenly in the adult years to produce a heart attack or gangrene of a leg, depending on the artery involved.

2 | CHOLESTEROL FUNDAMENTALS

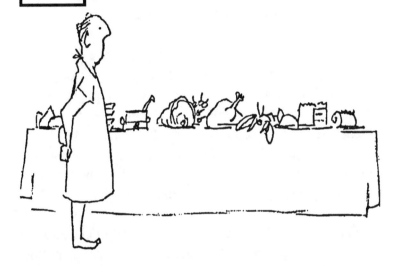

SURVIVAL STRATEGIES IN A WORLD OF ABUNDANCE

D espite its bad press, cholesterol is essential to full health. All tissues of the body use it as a cell wall and structural stabilizer. It stiffens and strengthens components, enabling them to function properly and withstand the pressures of their neighbors. At the molecular level it can be imagined to act like a chunk of chicken wire.

73

Cholesterol is an oil, however, and it must circulate in the water medium of blood so it must be wrapped in protein to keep it dissolved. When dissolved in the blood in excess it can penetrate the fine, porous lining of the artery walls and form deposits of waxy lumps called atheroma.

Thus we have a state of equilibrium in existence throughout life between cholesterol in the blood flowing through the arteries and its deposits under the linings. The greater the concentration of cholesterol in the blood, the greater the tendency for the deposits to form. Conversely, the lower the concentration of cholesterol in the blood, the lesser the tendency for deposits to form and the greater the tendency for those that are already there to regress or go away.

Healthy heart and brain arteries are soft and flexible. They are about as big around on average as a pencil, hollow tubes of muscle that work to deliver the heart's outpourings, a recycled 3500 gallons of blood a day. The heart pumps and the arteries help speed the blood along a vast delivery network of capillaries, the tiniest of blood vessels, an estimated 400 miles of them in each pound of flesh.

Coronary artery disease has come to be a household term because it describes those arteries nearest the heart whose obstruction leads to sudden death. The name comes from corona, which describes how they go around the heart. When a coronary artery becomes stiff and plugs with the cholesterol of atheroma deposits, the heart is deprived of its own blood supply and it aches on effort or a patch of its muscle dies.

Deposits of cholesterol or atheroma are not uniform throughout the arterial tree, as with say, calcium deposits along a water pipe. Cholesterol deposits are chunky or irregular, tending to form in arteries at points of stretch or tension. And they occur throughout the body. When an individual has coronary artery disease, the process is not confined to the heart but affects the entire system. There is disease throughout the body, including the arteries of the brain and legs.

"CHOLESTEROL IS THE SINGLE MOST IMPORTANT ELEMENT IN THE HEART ATTACK PROBLEM, AND GETTING ITS BLOOD LEVELS DOWN IS ESSENTIAL"

All major studies give special significance to cholesterol in the development of coronary artery disease. It is the single most important element in the heart attack problem, and getting its blood levels down is essential. But other factors have been shown to contribute as well. A sedentary lifestyle (of less than three miles a week on foot) has been shown to be a heart attack risk factor. Cigarette smoking too.   Obesity of over 25 pounds, especially around the waist; an elevated blood pressure, or blood triglyceride or blood sugar. All are risk factors for coronary artery disease but blood cholesterol tops the list.

Coronary artery narrowing is still an uncommon disorder among people whose daily calories come predominantly from wheat, rice or corn; or whose daily lives call for heavy expenditures of effort. Heart patients are usually sedentary males. And at the table they prefer their corn to have been fed first to cattle for conversion into the 200 pounds of animal tissue we eat every year. The distribution of heart disease across Europe is highest in the northern countries, lowest in the southern, and intermediate in those between. This correlates well with intakes of flesh, cheese and butter in the north, and of grains, fruits, and vegetables in the south.

During this century it has become much easier to get sick with coronary artery disease than to avoid it;   to choose eating and living patterns of maximum convenience and minimal restraint. *If you are signing up people who would like to dine first class regularly and play the flute forever, please place my name at the top of your list,* most of us would say. So far, however, it looks impossible. We live in a harsher kind of world.

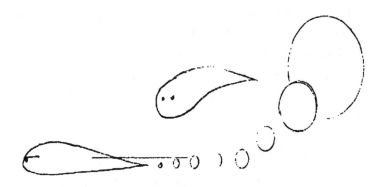

Once in the blood, cholesterol circulates in two major forms that should be of special interest to anyone concerned about heart health. Because they were originally separated by centrifugation in the laboratory they have been identified by their densities, i.e. whether high density or low density. And because cholesterol is a fat, an oil, it must be solubilized in the blood with a protein wrapper, a lipoprotein. The "bad," or potentially injurious form, is called LDL (Low Density Lipoprotein) cholesterol. This is the cholesterol transport form that tends to be deposited in tissues leading to its accumulation in the arteries and to heart attacks.

The "good" cholesterol is called HDL (High Density Lipoprotein) cholesterol. It does not tend to be deposited in the tissues but rather it is delivered to the liver for

77

secretion in the bile and eventual excretion into the digestive tract and out of the body. And since high levels of HDL cholesterol have been shown to be associated with fewer heart attacks, studies have been undertaken on ways to get HDL levels as high as possible. All point to exercise as the best way.

"ALL STUDIES HAVE INDICATED THAT SIGNIFICANT PROTECTION FROM HEART ATTACKS BEGINS WITH HDL CHOLESTEROL LEVELS ABOVE 50 MG %. "

One report from Houston concerned a population of men in a variety of situations of mobility and immobility to study the effects of exercise on their HDL levels. Paralyzed men had the lowest levels, marathoners had the highest and sedentary office workers were in between. Heart attack preventive HDL levels are above 50 mg. %. Men who were immobilized with severe back injuries had HDL levels that average 35. Otherwise fit but sedentary men averaged HDL levels of 45. Male runners who covered 10-15 miles a week had levels of 55, while those who were into distance running and covered 40-50 miles a week had heart protection levels of 65 mg. %. All studies have indicated that significant protection from heart attacks begins with HDL cholesterol levels above 50 mg.%.

Up to the menopause, women generally have higher levels of HDL cholesterol than men, thanks to the influence of their sex hormones. This helps account for women tending to be protected from coronary artery disease up to the menopause. Taking estrogens after the menopause helps to maintain the HDL at their previous heart protective levels.

Back to the other kind, the LDL "bad" cholesterol...it's the package that delivers cholesterol to all the tissues. It can be lowered best by changes in one's food habits already mentioned, a decreased consumption of animal and dairy fats and a decrease in dietary cholesterol itself. So keep the two cholesterols separate in your thinking, forget risk ratios. Keep the total with its large LDL fraction down with good food habits, and keep the HDL up with good fitness habits.

LEGS ARE NOT VESTIGIAL ORGANS

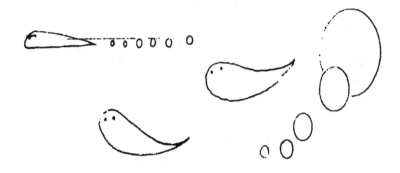

B ut there's another kind of fat in the blood that also narrows arteries. It's not the problem that cholesterol is, but it can be a problem. Called triglyceride, it is a different kind of fat than cholesterol. Triglycerides are not constructed like the chicken wire cholesterol molecule. They are similar in construction to the oils used in cooking and the oils that make up butter and lard. In small amounts they circulate in the blood as supplies of fat for energy. In excess, they accumulate in the arteries just like LDL cholesterol.

The debate over whether high triglyceride levels contribute to heart disease has been answered in the affirmative. When elevated cholesterol levels are allowed for and they often complicate elevated triglyceride levels high triglycerides in and of themselves have a distinctive and bad effect on artery hardening. The most common cause of an elevated triglyceride level is an elevated cholesterol, where it acts like the tail of the cholesterol kite, but some patients have isolated elevated levels. For them weight control may be the only element in their life that needs to be changed.

Other individuals are uniquely sensitive to the effect of alcohol and for them, stopping drinking lowers their triglycerides. Others are susceptible to high intakes of refined starches or sugars. For these reasons high triglyceride patients are often advised to control their weight, reduce or eliminate alcohol, and keep their sugar and refined starch intakes low. In addition, some ocean fish or their oils have been shown to markedly lower triglyceride levels.

So the HDL cholesterol is an exercise function, what about the total cholesterol? It's a combination of HDL and LDL and it's a food function. Two nutrients drive it up and one helps keep it down. Fiber helps keep cholesterol down by capturing it in the gut and preventing its uptake. The two nutrients that send cholesterol up are cholesterol in food itself and saturated fats and oils. These two items make such major contributions to today's food preferences that major cultural and commercial pressures are at work resisting change. But change we must, *and that means eating less red meat and less chicken and less fish, too. Because they are all major sources of cholesterol.*

FITNESS FEEDINGS

CLEAN SHOPPING

Choose products low in fat or fat-free. In the dairy department this means selecting skim milk, skim milk yogurt, and skim milk cottage cheese.

Try to steer clear of cheese. Even those claiming to be low fat are too high in fat and salt. If you love cheese, use sprinkle cheeses, hard pungent cheeses such as Feta, Romano, Parmesan or Sapsego on your dishes. The fat and salt content is high in these cheeses, but little is needed for flavor.

Intact fish, turkey and chicken are the tissues of choice. Intact means not ground up, not breaded, and not butterballed. They also have less saturated fat than beef or pork, but they all contain cholesterol. Avoid cold cuts and sausage.

Be wary of products made of 100% vegetable oil, and often loudly proclaiming their freedom from cholesterol on their labels. If the vegetable oil is co-conut or palm, it is a saturated oil.

On food labels, add 0 to the fat grams to translate their contribution to the caloies, thus 5 gms. = 50 calories.

COACH'S CORNER

A LITTLE BRAN ON THE SIDE

For the average American man the likely reason for his next hospital admission will be coronary artery disease. Yet heart attacks were rare in the early decades of this century. They've turned out to be the result of a cholesterol problem which has turned out to be the result of a nutrition problem. Blood cholesterol levels are too high, thanks to our diet, not to our physical inactivity.

The Anticoronary Club of New York has been doing something about this for more than 45 years. It is an association of coronary artery disease patients organized to test the notion that lowering blood cholesterol levels by dietary means would reduce the ravages of coronary heart disease, and it does. Their message is that we must lower food fat and food cholesterol, and increase our intakes of food fiber.

High fiber diets can produce marked losses of cholesterol from the digestive tract beginning after only 4 days. Diets that are naturally high in fiber work best, rather than breakfast bran supplements. But studies have shown that just switching from breakfast bran to rolled oats can produce a 35% increase in losses of cholesterol from the digestive tract.

3 | FATS AND OILS FUNDAMENTALS

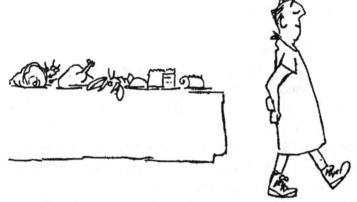

WHAT'S FOOD GOT TO DO WITH CANCER?

We've been adjusting to cancer-causing agents called carcinogens over eons of time. Most plants, for example, make potential carcinogens as natural pesticides to defend themselves against insect predators. Up to 10% of the dry weight of plants is toxic defensive chemical weaponry. The caffeine of coffee is a good example. It's a pesticide against predator bugs. We eat plants in amounts that provide us with an annual carcinogen exposure measured in pounds yet we've lived with these exposures a long time with no apparent ill effects. We've also lived a long time with natural, anti-cancer dietary defenses. And their loss or reduction leave us vulnerable. This development so alarmed a group of scientists a few years ago that they did a public about face on the safety of the American diet.

"We know more now," said the chairman at his press conference, explaining the committee's U-turn from a previous reassuring report on diet and disease. He was responding to a reporter's unfriendly question about the recommendations of a previous committee of the National Academy of Science which, in 1982, had reassured us there was no need to be concerned about our diet. The new committee now reported otherwise.

The 1982 report had rattled the nutrition community with its assurances that our diet was the envy of the world. There was no good evidence linking it to major diseases. Very reassuring, almost. But journalistic revelations on the heels of the report indicated that the most influential committee members had food industry ties which made their reassurances suspect. The new committee told us to cut the fat and double the fiber.

To back off for a moment...cancer kills more than 20% of all adult Americans. It develops in any given tissue through a succession of steps over a period of about 10 years, before being recognized clinically, then in the average individual it kills by spread over the next 10 years, almost in spite of whatever is done.

In humans, the cervix has provided opportunities to study these steps in the evolution of cancer. The first stage is dysplasia ... the development of a collection of abnormal cells. They come and go over the years, developing and receding, and they may never go any further, but if cancer is to develop they persist and go on to the second stage, still not officially cancer.

The cells in the second stage show no tendency to invade their neighborhood (which is a cancer behavior hallmark) but they look more sinister under the microscope, more abnormal. This stage is called cancer-in-place. Both stage one and stage two are being followed in long-term trials underway all over the world. In New York City, one effort is evaluating the benefits of Vitamin A supplements. Early laboratory studies have shown cancer-blocking properties for the vitamin, the same vitamin necessary for normal vision and fighting infections. It takes part in chemical reactions that influence the duplication of cells: Normalizing cell duplication and preventing invasion or cancer stage three.

The third and final step to full cancer is invasion. Cells no longer respect tissue boundaries and grow everywhere. They also keep duplicating themselves, having escaped the usual limits on life span. They are both immortal and amoral, because normal cells die.

Whether in the cervix or the bowel or the lung, normal cells live within the boundaries of their neighborhoods. They grow old and after a certain number of duplications, they die, programmed to behave this way genetically. In turning cancerous this control is lost, and new research suggests that the immortality of cancerous cells results from very minor alterations in their genetic material, perhaps as little as a single amino acid. Such alterations may be provoked by environmental triggers such as chronic irritation, or by carcinogens like saccharine or sunshine. Such alterations may be prevented by particular nutrients.

By studying the application of Vitamin A to this process, it's hoped that stages leading to cancer can be interrupted. It will not be a swift unraveling. Keep in mind that Vitamin A can poison in doses only three or four times above the daily requirement, so don't take Vitamin A supplements except for the small amount that's in the standard multiple vitamin pill. There are safer alternatives, also being studied around the world.

Researchers in New Jersey have found that vegetable consumption provides protection against lung cancer. In a case-controlled study, the greatest protection was provided by dark or yellow-orange vegetables. Consumption of fruits did not appear to be protective, nor did taking vitamin supplements, but a good vegetable intake somehow prevented the critical events that lead to cancer production, even in two-pack a day smokers. It is one of several studies demonstrating a protective effect of diet on cigarette smokers. Indeed, in the past 25 years more than 300 studies have confirmed relationships, positive and negative on cancer.

> *"OF PARTICULAR ADDITIONAL INTEREST ... WAS THE FINDING THAT A HIGH FIBER DIET WAS ONLY PROTECTIVE WHEN VEGETABLES PROVIDED THE FIBER."*

Cancer of the colon is another very common cancer. It too can be influenced by diet. A recent report from Australia on more than 700 cases occurring since 1980, confirmed that fiber and fat had their recognized effects; the more fat in the diet the greater likelihood of cancer; the more fiber in the diet the lesser the likelihood of cancer.

FATS AND OILS CONSUMPTION IN GRAMS
AND COLON CANCER DEATHS

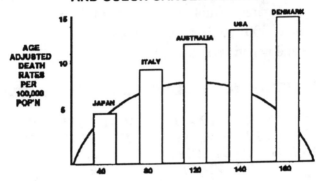

AGE
ADJUSTED
DEATH
RATES
PER
100,000
POP'N

JAPAN, ITALY, AUSTRALIA, USA, DENMARK

**DAILY CONSUMPTION: FROM A RICE SOCIETY TO
DAIRIES AND MEAT**

Of particular additional interest to the Australian researchers, echoing the New Jersey observations, was the finding that a high-fiber diet was only protective when vegetables provided the fiber. Grain fiber was not protective, nor was fruit fiber, nor beans, nuts or seed fiber. Just vegetables. And among those especially protective were the cruciferous vegetables: cauliflower, cabbage, broccoli and brussel sprouts. So a vegetable switch at sweet roll time may be the smartest, if eccentric, anti-cancer move you ever made.

Both breast and colon cancers are common cancers. New York researchers report that among 1,000 cases of breast cancer there was three times more colon cancer than one would find in the general population. Out in California, breast cancer researchers have been following their own food and cancer trail, studying droplets of fluid collected from the breasts of women attending a cancer screening clinic in San Francisco. The researchers were looking for abnormal or precancerous cells, and they found them to be associated with chronic constipation.

Of the women studied to date, those who reported a habit of constipation (having only one or two bowel movements a week) were more likely to have fibrocystic or nodular breasts. This is postulated to result from prolonged contact between digestive products and bacteria in the intestinal tract which are known to produce chemicals that promote cancer. The researchers found that correction of the constipation led to improvement in cells being excreted from the breasts. Less constipation meant fewer disordered breast cells.

Back in 1980, thousands of registered nurses aged 34 to 50 years old who, as far as they knew, were free of cancer, enrolled in a long-term cancer study. They completed a questionnaire designed to measure their daily consumption of fat and other nutrients. Those in the highest fat intake group consumed 44% of their calories as fat. Over the next decade of follow-up more than 600 cases of breast cancer occurred among the nurses studied. No difference has been demonstrated between those on lower fat intake "low fat" benefit, and the negative findings have received much public attention: fat intake played no role in breast cancer. A more correct conclusion, however, is that there's no benefit in reducing fat intake from 44% to 34%. Because there is probably no difference. Cutting to 30% is an empty effort as laboratory animal studies have shown. Both 30% and 38% are overloads. As a general rule for the reader, get to 20% by halving your fat intake. Avoiding cancer is a real prospect from dietary changes involving less fat and more fiber, but not from token gestures.

FATS AND OILS CONSUMPTION IN GRAMS AND BREAST CANCER DEATHS

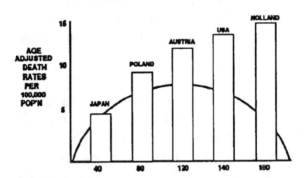

DAILY CONSUMPTION: FROM A RICE SOCIETY TO DAIRIES AND MEAT

I n Italy, where the population is reasonably homogeneous, there are two different fat and fiber eating styles - Northern and Southern. The North is affluent and industrial; the South less affluent and more agricultural. Northern Italian eating is high in fat and dairy based; the Southern diet is low in fat and vegetable-based. In a recent confirmation of the breast cancer dietary fat association, scientists in Milan correlated increased breast cancer death rates in the North with the increased consumption of high-fat foods such as milk and cheese. There was less breast cancer in the South with their vegetables and pastas. Indeed, death rates from all cancers were found to be higher in the North than the South, a regional food story with implications for us all.

"HALF OF ALL OF TODAY'S CANCERS ARE DIET-ASSOCIATED OR DIET-MODIFIED."

Food habits known to reduce the risk of developing breast cancer are low in fat and high in fiber so researchers in Hawaii are re-evaluating their own efforts in the management of established breast cancer in a population of cancerous women. Prior to developing their cancers, the women in the study ate mainstream American: 45% of their calories from fats and oils, 40% from carbohydrates and 15% from protein. They also had low intakes of fiber.

After the usual surgical and medical treatment of their breast cancers, the women were placed on low-fat, high-fiber diets. A vegetarian diet, in fact, that provided less than 10% of the day's calories from fat, about 12% from protein and 80% from complex carbohydrates. It contained four times more fiber than their previous diets. Compliance by the patients, many of whom were ethnic Japanese and culturally attuned to more vegetables, has been excellent. They have shown swift reduction in biological indicators associated with breast cancer: their obesity, their blood cholesterol, and certain hormone levels. All the data improved. The cancer-promoting internal environment of these women has been changed for the better, and preliminary reports indicate the beginning of a survival separation when compared to non-diet-intervention controls.

Cancer growth and spread, once established, has been found to be encouraged by the same factors that promote its appearance originally. There are implications in these observations for individuals who have cancer and undergone appropriate medical management. Changes in food habits still hold prospect of benefit for them in terms of prolonging survival or minimizing recurrence.

Aggrieved producers of fat-laden foods will feel unfairly fingered in the education process that must follow these discoveries. They may even deceive themselves on the insignificant contribution made by their own particular product to the collective problem, and they have already begun to defend themselves in their ads. It's important, however, that we not let them deceive us as well. The results are in: half of all of today's cancers are diet-associated or diet-modified.

WHOLE FOOD IS USER - FRIENDLY

FITNESS FEEDINGS

CLEAN TREATS:
PEACH OR APPLE STRUDEL

4 sheets phyllo dough
1 T lemon juice
 Pam
2 T brown sugar
1/3 cup bread crumbs
1 T flour
2 cups sliced peaches, peeled

Spray one sheet of dough with Pam, lay on a dish towel, and sprinkle with bread crumbs. Repeat with next two sheets, laying one on the other, (last sheet needs no Pam). Mix peaches, sugar, flour and lemon juice together and heap along the long side to within 1-1/2" of edges and one end. Roll up carefully and place on Pammed baking sheet. Tuck in ends. Brush with 1 tsp margarine. Bake at 375 degrees for 45 minutes or until golden.

Substitute 2 cups sliced apples in above recipe and add if desired: 3/4 tsp cinnamon, pinch nutmeg, 1/4 cup raisins.

COACH'S CORNER

THINK CRUCIFEROUS

One of the most notable food changes among the Japanese since 1950 is their increased consumption of fats and oils; more meat and animal products and far greater use of vegetable oils in their cooking. This food change has been paralleled by a striking increase in deaths from cancer of the prostate among Japanese men, and cancer of the breast in Japanese women.

A relationship between high fat intakes and cancer promotion has been established by dozens of studies in other population groups, as well as in the laboratory. When breast tumors are implanted into cancer-free mice, for instance, the cancer grows best if the animal is on a high fat diet.

Cancer control begins by eating less fat, and continues by eating more fibered foods and more vegetables. Members of the cruciferous vegetable family (cabbage, cauliflower, broccoli and brussels sprouts) are also especially protective.

4 | SALT FUNDAMENTALS

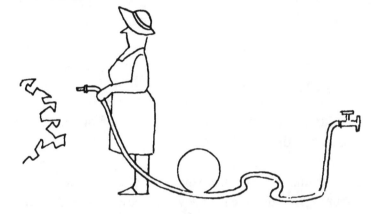

HOW'S SALT RELATED TO HIGH BLOOD PRESSURE?

F or any pressure to be developed and sustained in a closed system like the circulation, one needs a pump (the heart), and a distribution network of pipes or tubes (the arteries and veins).

Essentially the cycle runs like this: Blood that is rich in oxygen from the lungs is pumped through the heart and out into a system of ever narrowing passageways, then into a mesh of billions of microscopic tubes called capillaries. At the point of narrowing, where the passageways become a mesh, nozzles of muscle cuffs are located. They help maintain pressure throughout the system like the nozzle on a garden hose; the tighter or the more closed, the higher the pressure.

Once through the system, blood travels back to the heart in widening passageways of veins. Now it contains waste or carbon dioxide and upon reaching the heart it is pumped into the lungs for purification. And so on and on, recycling thousands of gallons of blood a day.

What determines blood pressure in the system is not the heart-pump, nor the great and visible arteries and veins, but the billions of tiny and invisible blood vessels at the very end of the arterial line. The walls of these smallest arteries, just before becoming capillaries contain the muscle cuffs that create the nozzles that effect the flow of blood and raise the pressure. Open, they increase flow and lower the blood pressure. Thus, the greatest effect on blood pressure is made not by influencing the pump as much as by influencing the nozzles. Dietary salt acts as a constricting agent on the small blood vessel cuffs in susceptible individuals. In young people, high dietary salt intakes usually have no effect on the blood pressure. Their systems can clear the excess and prevent the pressure from rising. That capacity to clear the huge amounts of salt in our diet -more than five times what we need - is eventually lost by late adult life in half of the American population, so they develop high blood pressure.

In our distant past, it was the job of our kidneys to prevent a loss of sodium from the system. In evolutionary terms, we carried a marine internal environment into a dry, low-salt environment so we developed our blood pressure controlling skills in an environment very different from today's. It was low in salt and high in potassium. Today it's the reverse. Today's high sodium low potassium diet eventually overwhelms the kidneys. It's a shabby way to treat two loyal, hard-working friends.

"OUR PREFERENCE FOR PROCESSED FOODS MEANS THAT POTASSIUM LEVELS IN OUR DIET DECLINE, WHILE SODIUM GOES HIGH."

Potassium in food has a countering effect on this influence of salt or sodium. A high potassium intake from a diet rich in fruits and vegetables has a neutralizing effect on the blood pressure tendencies of excessive sodium. But our preference for processed foods means that potassium levels in our diet decline, while sodium goes high. It's a double whammy that promotes high blood pressure. Other factors are involved but over the long haul, salt has proven to be a major contributor to high blood pressure and that's bad news because it can provoke a stroke in one of two ways; from a clot or from bleeding. A bleeding episode is the more dramatic disaster. It comes about because of ballooning and weakening of the wall, like inflating an inner tube outside a tire. Over a period of time - about 20 years - the weakness develops from a bulge to a burst that can cause an immediate and often fatal stroke from brain hemorrhage.

In addition to the burst and bleed, high blood pressure is also associated with an excessive accumulation of cholesterol in the walls of the arteries of the heart and brain. This process narrows arteries down and can, before a burst elsewhere, lead to a plugging. In the heart, it's a heart attack and in the brain, it's a stroke.

RISK OF DEVELOPING A HEART ATTACK WITH HIGH BLOOD PRESSURE

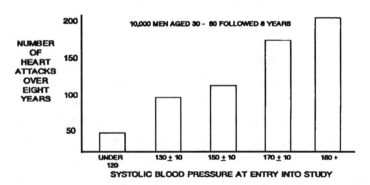

H igh blood pressure eventually leads to problems that are lethal after years of being quietly and painlessly elevated. It is a sneaky disorder that affects almost a third of Americans, especially Black Americans. Recent surveys indicate that the blood pressures of black Americans are not as much a consequence of their high salt intakes as their low potassium intakes.

"HIGH BLOOD PRESSURE IS A SNEAKY DISORDER THAT AFFECTS ALMOST A THIRD OF AMERICANS, ESPECIALLY BLACK AMERICANS."

Because Black Americans are especially susceptible to high blood pressure, their particular food changes over this century are instructive. Compared to their diet from the turn of the century, they are getting at least as much salt but probably half the potassium. The hard-time foods of greens, grits and sweet potatoes which are naturally high in potassium and low in salt have given way to the good-time foods of corn flakes, chips and fast foods, which are low in potassium and high in salt. This sharp reduction in their potassium intake may have especially sensitized them to the stroke-promoting effects of sodium. It's a possibility

103

all Americans ought to consider, especially those among us with a family history of hypertension or strokes.

Potassium occurs naturally in our diet in fresh fruits and vegetables as well as in whole-grain cereals and cereal products. Potassium consumption by Americans has been declining over this century for two reasons. One results from food processing which leads to potassium losses (and sadly to sodium additives). A second decline is the result of our reduced intake of calories. Excess body weight is now a national problem, so we have begun to cut back on calories, currently eating 30-40% fewer than we did at the turn of the century. So our total potassium intake is reduced by most estimates to about half what it was 75 years ago.

HEALTH IS AN INSIDE JOB

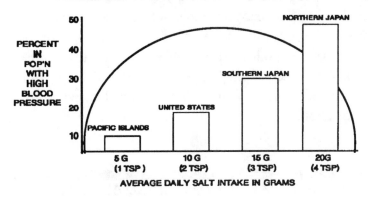

PREVALENCE OF HIGH BLOOD PRESSURE
RELATIONSHIP TO AVERAGE DAILY INTAKE OF SALT

O utside this country there are blood pressure lessons to be learned from around the world. Sweden has provided completely free health care to its citizens for more than 50 years, yet an active alternative health movement exists in that country as it does here. The movement promotes self care through lifestyle change and emphasizes prevention through the management of disorders such as high cholesterol and blood pressure. In a nation where health services and medicines are free one might expect little interest in a "health yourself" message but such is not the case.

A total of 29 adult Swedes who were on medication an average of eight years for their hypertension decided to try low-salt, vegetarian diets for a year. Side effects from the medication had become intolerable so they stopped their drugs, ate no salt, no animal products, eggs or dairy products. For other reasons they took no tea, coffee or chocolate; they wanted to return to natural living. In all participants blood pressures fell to levels that called for no medication.

"PEOPLE MAY BE CONCERNED ABOUT THEIR HEALTH BUT THE FIRST THING THEY WANT IS FLAVOR."

In 30 studies of human populations over the past 50 years, researchers have found close correlations between salt consumption and high blood pressure levels: The higher the intake the higher the pressure. In Belgium, for example, where a reduced salt intake was promoted nationally from 1970 to 1980, a fall in daily salt consumption from three to two teaspoons a day was associated with a significant fall in deaths from stroke.

In a new low-salt soup line, Campbell has used spices, herbs and wines to make the best-tasting, low-sodium soups possible, but sales are only slightly above those of

106

the old line. "If we're making any money, " said a spokesman," it isn't very much. People may be concerned about their health but the first thing they want is flavor." It's not going to be an easy transition, if it occurs at all.

Intensive public education campaigns in Finland, Belgium and Australia indicate that while individuals can be taught the benefits of restricting salt, in the collective or as populations, they rarely can be persuaded to go beyond the simple step of not adding it at the table. We like our salt when hypertension and its consequences are but a dim and distant prospect.

NOTHING WORKS IF YOU DON'T

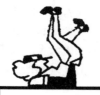

FITNESS FEEDINGS

SOME SALT SUBSTITUTES FOR SEASONING

BAY LEAF- the familiar taste of bay leaf is found in bean recipes and Italian dishes. Try it with chicken, fish, green beans, carrots, beets, eggplant, onions, white potatoes, summer squash, tomatoes.

OREGANO- both oregano and basil give pizza and spaghetti sauce their familiar taste. Try oregano with chicken, green beans, broccoli, cabbage, carrots, cauliflower, onions, peas, white potatoes, spinach, tomatoes, turnips.

GINGER-a familiar taste found in Chinese stir-fry. Try it with chicken, fish, carrots, cauliflower, beets, onions, sweet potatoes, winter squash.

BASIL-try it with green beans,cabbage, corn, eggplant, onions, peas, white potatoes, spinach, summer squash, winter squash, tomatoes.

COACH'S CORNER

SODIUM'S YOUR PROBLEM

It's the sodium part of salt that does the damage. The effects of sharp reductions of sodium in individuals with established high blood pressure have been well documented.They are "cured" of their high blood pressure if they get their intakes low enough. Sodium may be an essential mineral in our diet, but the amounts that we consume are at least 10 times beyond what we need.

Twenty to thirty percent of Americans are predisposed to develop high blood pressure as they age, in the presence of an intake of sodium as high as the one we consume. By the simple maneuver of eliminating salt at the table and in the kitchen we can cut our intakes in half, but that is still not a low salt diet.

A daily intake that is truly controlled means no fast foods, no convenience foods and no packaged foods. It means much more self-cooking. It means more food label reading. In fact, a watch must be kept on everything eaten as well as certain liquids especially diet pop. It is a tough program to follow today because it means returning to diet of fresh fruits, vegetables, whole grain breads and cereals, fresh fish, chicken, lean meat, and home-prepared foods.

5 STRESS FUNDAMENTALS

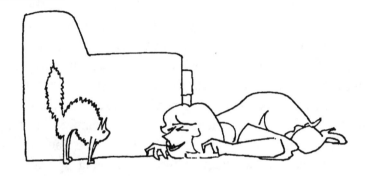

AM I STRESSED OR JUST HIGH STRUNG?

F or hundreds of thousands of years our species coped with stress and didn't know it. We'd have called it responding physically and emotionally to threats. The older, more primitive part of the human brain evolved to equip us with speedy reflex responses to a threatening world, a world where the primary object of existence was to find a meal without becoming someone else's. The reactions that evolved to serve this survival need were not thoughtful, reasoned or deliberate, but quick and direct.

They ensured survival through fight or flight, attack or avoid. In today's world the moods that are part of these reactions are called expressions of biostress.

Preparations for fight or flight begin reflexively and immediately. They require no thought and no conscious participation. They do not involve New Brain, that recent and sophisticated part of the brain that makes us human and the most intelligent of earth's creatures. When threats are perceived they activate Old Brain's reflexes. (Old Brain is millions of years old. It is a legacy we share with many creatures. It is about the size of your closed hand and is located under New Brain at the top of your spinal cord. New Brain grew out of Old Brain fairly recently, and in any crisis Old Brain reflexively gets involved. It has been our lifeguard too long to stay on the sidelines). These reflexes set up a brief electrical response phase to be followed by a sustained and powerful chemical phase. It's a sequenced series of preparations that trigger one or a combination of two moods: fear or anger.

The electrical phase of the alarm reaction, is the startle reflex; the jump to full alert. The chemical phase of adrenalin follows close behind this agent of flight or fight and its moods of fear or anger. In large amounts it's the hormone of panic, in small amounts the hormone of challenge, of get up and go. Adrenalin gets the body's tissues into shape for action. It stops the secretion of juices in the gut, keeping fluids in the blood to better nerve the muscles; hence the dry mouth. It shunts blood from the skin to flight-fight muscles; hence the pallor. It secretes scent signals of danger to other members of the tribe; hence the heavy sweating of armpits, palms and soles. It tones up the delivery of blood to the muscles; hence the elevated blood pressure and heart rate. And it heightens nervous system preparation for action; hence the alertness, agitation, restlessness and trembling.

But in today's world such behavior is usually unsettling and inappropriate. The threats we experience are seldom physical and rarely life threatening...an unexpected expense, a family quarrel, a work dispute or traffic gridlock. We respond to them all the same way, as though they were physical threats. Old Brain sets up its ancient alarms and the body responds as though one's life were on the line. In a civilized world we must check these built-in flight-fight impulses and moods, control that reflex biology. Prepared for action, however, and forced by social constraints to suppress it, we experience irritability, tension, inability to concentrate, stuttering and speech difficulties, trembling, digestive upsets, high blood pressure and headaches.

The normal circulation accomplishes what it's supposed to by coursing through billions of blood vessels invisible to the naked eye. The larger ones that we recognize as arteries and veins are not important blood pressure determinants. It's the tiniest ones at the microscopic level that can open and close that determine blood pressure. And stress signals sent from the brain release the adrenalin that causes the closing of the nozzles that raise the blood pressure.

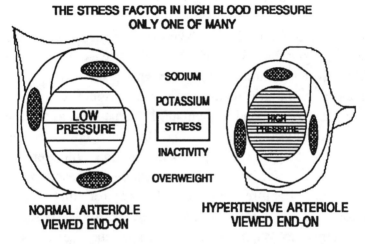

THE STRESS FACTOR IN HIGH BLOOD PRESSURE
ONLY ONE OF MANY

SODIUM

POTASSIUM

STRESS

INACTIVITY

OVERWEIGHT

LOW PRESSURE

HIGH PRESSURE

NORMAL ARTERIOLE VIEWED END-ON

HYPERTENSIVE ARTERIOLE VIEWED END-ON

ADRENALIN RELEASED FROM NERVE ENDINGS CAUSES THE BLOOD VESSEL NOZZLES TO TIGHTEN AND RAISE THE PRESSURE

Fit individuals usually spare themselves this spinning of their energy wheels, these expressions of biostress. Fit individuals have already undertaken the regular redistribution of their supplies of adrenalin. Their workouts release adrenalin from nerve endings to bathe their brains in it, lifting the mood and instilling confidence. The natural tone in their muscles is down, their blood pressure is down, and their systems are relaxed even if on full alert from alarm signals. How so? Well, within 10 minutes of any brisk walk or jog or workout, adrenalin begins to be released from these nerve endings: its levels rise in the blood and bathe the brain in energy and confidence. As long as the workout continues, adrenalin continues to be released and to benefit the brain.

The executive washroom has provided researchers an opportunity to confirm the adrenalin response to stress. The washroom offered a workday environment to collect executive urine and measure adrenalin byproducts in it, a reliable chemical measure of the day's level of stress. Fit executives were found to put out only half as much adrenalin in the course of their stressful days as did their sedentary colleagues. In the sedentary or unfit individual, adrenalin that had not been pre-released but remained stored up in nerve endings was reflexively dumped during periods of stress. Muscle fibers became tightened or vibrated fitfully, twitching ineffectively while the leaked adrenalin sent alarm into all the tissues. Regular adrenalin transfer through fitness is the best kept secret of biostress management.

"...A CHRONIC, FRUSTATED STATE OF READINESS FOR PHYSICAL ACTION THAT'S SELDOM TAKEN."

Beyond the assumption underlying the above comments, that we all respond to threats the same way and would benefit from a daily workout is the everyday observation that some of us are more easily stressed than others, that there are personality factors in play here as well.

Researchers into personality and its development continue to separate the role of heredity and environment on our attitudes and behavior. Are we what we are from nature or nurture?

A major finding in these researches over the past decade is that the environment shared by members of a family plays a surprisingly small role in producing family member similarities. Working with identical twins (who have identical genes) raised together and raised apart, researchers continue to produce evidence that genetic similarity is as good a predictor of personality as is the environment in which the individual was raised.

Genes or heredity seem to account for at least 50% of behavior traits in any given population. That's the inherited wiring in our brain. The remaining 50% comes from environmental influences that are unique to each person's experience, such as parent-child interactions, peer influences, teachers and random events.

The measurement of one's personality, however, is itself a controversial topic. There is general agreement among researchers that we all have two personality "super factors." One of these is our Extroversion which covers sociability and the general level of impulsiveness. The other is our Neuroticism which covers emotional sensitivity and the general level of anxiety or susceptibility to stress. Both of these "super factors" are present in every personality but to varying degrees. There's no agreement as yet among the scientists on how a normal personality divides them up. In addition, other factors play modifying roles, factors such as one's sense of well-being, social effectiveness, degree of achievement, alienation, aggression, traditionalism, risk-avoidance, self-control, etc. All these factors are recognizable components of anyone's personality, and all are being studied long-term by researchers working with identical twins. Their aim is a better understanding of nature and nurture. Are you easily angered because of how you are put together or how you were treated at a tender age?

The very nature of the research forces scientists studying twins to rely on much questioning and subjectivity. There are few hard end points as in physics or chemistry. As a result they often quibble about each other's techniques and approaches, but their results over the past decade have put them in general agreement that the environment shared by a family plays a surprisingly minor role in the formation of personality.

It comes as no surprise to most parents. They have already discovered how previous relatives' characteristics reappear in their kids. Animal breeders too, who produce products for markets as varied as the bull ring, the farmyard or domestic petdome, breed creatures for temperament as well as structural characteristics. Breeders know that genes influence the personalities of their products and they have acted upon that knowledge for centuries. They can and do selectively breed for intensity of emotional response and thresholds of arousal; race horses versus riding horses.

What these observations mean with regard to stress management is that everyone has varying degrees of susceptibility to the same sets of inputs. There are skittish race horses and there are phlegmatic workhorses. What could be a simple disturbance to one, produces panic in another. In human terms, the latter individual, by the very nature of his or her genes must play the game differently, at times having the foresight to decline to play.

 tress is a pain, a mood pain and usually not a physical pain, but still a pain. And because avoiding pain is a law of life, stress produces unpleasant feelings to avoid or to be rid of it. It's a mood that evolved to drive us to seek relief. Some turn to calming chemicals; smoking, alcohol or drugs. A recent Australian study of alcohol and high blood pressure was instructive. Although not usually regarded as a lifestyle component or even a nutrient, alcohol does provide from 10% to 20% of the day's calories to regular drinkers, and it can also play a role in their blood pressure levels.

The Australians found that drinking more than six servings a day had a serious compromising effect on attempts to control high blood pressure even with strong medication. They persuaded the heavy drinkers to reduce their consumption to two servings a day for a period of six months; and simple alcohol limitation alone lowered all their measurements. They concluded that the benefits of any blood pressure medication or any dietary change in the face of continued heavy drinking is seriously compromised or ineffective in most patients.

"DRINKING MORE THAN SIX SERVINGS A DAY HAD SERIOUS COMPROMISING EFFECT ON ATTEMPTS TO CONTROL HIGH BLOOD PRESSURE EVEN WITH STRONG MEDICATION."

Unless properly managed, biostress phenomena can lead to a chronic frustrated state of readiness for physical action that's seldom taken. Addictive substances give a momentary relief from the frustrations but carry penalizing consequences. Managing biostress phenomena is about managing emotional energy, managing it in a way that harnesses its adrenalin for the day's objectives. The moods being managed are the moods of anger or anxiety, and they are energetic or action moods, thanks to the energy of adrenalin. Learning to manage anger means learning to manage adrenalin, before during and after perceived threats. Learning to manage tension and fear also means learning to manage adrenalin.

L ife is more stressful today than it was a hundred years ago in part because we lack the opportunity to work off the natural responses to everyday upsets. We don't use up the day's adrenalin stock anymore. In the time of human existence before this century, just getting through each day was physically demanding. It called up the adrenalin so that worry and aggravation, adrenalin's psychological components, were well blunted or worked off. Many relationships were saved in the days when wives could beat carpets and husbands chop wood.

Beyond being sedentary and out of shape, other body changes set the stage for increased susceptibility to feelings of stress, there are the physical changes like a hangover, the debility of illness, simple exhaustion, or the menopause.

Women into the menopause often complain of mood swings: episodes of irritability or depression with or without the sweats and skin flushing of hot flashes. What bothers most patients about their menopause is their nervousness, tension, insomnia and mood swings. The usual medical treatment for hot flashes consists of hormones which help stabilize the system. A regular walking program would help, too.

"...PUT ENOUGH ELASTICITY INTO YOUR DAILY EMOTIONAL TONE TO TAKE UPSETS AND AGGRAVATIONS IN STRIDE."

Whatever the triggering circumstances of the moods of stress, a variety of self-defense home measures are available that involve food and fitness changes. All can help unwind the nervous system and put enough elasticity into the daily emotional tone that one takes upsets and aggravations in stride. First of all, cut back on nervous system stimulants such as caffeine. It stimulates the brain, increases wakefulness and promotes excitability. In large doses it can cause panic attacks, twitching and convulsions. The same cutback applies to the nicotine of cigarettes. It too is a nervous system stimulant. Indeed, given intravenously it can cause convulsions. By continuing to impose these chemical stimulators on a tense nervous

121

system, you can snap the toughest tissue into irritable disarray.

Cut back too on sugar, as in refined sugar, and even fruit juices. Sugar is sharply absorbed from the digestive system. It spikes to high levels in the blood, stimulating an over-production of insulin. The insulin then over-reduces blood sugar levels so that after taking sugar, hypoglycemia can occur, adding its own contribution to irritability, trembling and tension. Start eating whole food: fruit and not juice, whole grain breads and cereals and not sweet rolls or sugared breakfast flakes.

Without question, stress gets the circulation rolling. It tones us up with adrenalin and readies the body for action. A certain amount is essential to full health, and we call that challenge or excitement. Too much, however, can lead to headaches, ulcers, high blood pressure and ultimately, strokes. Learn your tolerance limits and take off their anger-anxiety edge with a soaking tub, bubble bath or sauna; a massage, a hug, even sex...a certain amount of relaxation is essential to full health.

COACH'S CORNER

GOOD STRESS, BAD STRESS

Eliminating stress from daily life would make our days boring. Stress is a very natural circumstance for us to live and thrive in. It stretches us. It keeps us toned. It puts interest and challenge and excitement into life. Those benefits have been described as "good stress," as compared to "bad stress."

So what is stress anyway? Well, its an unpleasant mood, one of anger (irritation or aggravation), or one of anxiety (deadlines or pressures). Both moods get us ready to take muscular defensive action.

The whole process is a legacy from a dim and distant past that once activated us to fight or flee (and still does), although we try to control such events. In small amounts, stress can be like mustard, livening things up. So rather than call the spice of stress "Good Stress", why not call it Challenge, and save the word stress for what it really is, a pain?

Any pain is too much and we each must learn to recognize what is excessive. Its an individual decision, where you strike a balance between the forces of too little and too much. So thumbs up for challenge and thumbs down on stress.

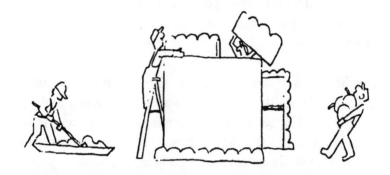

6 | LIFESTYLE FUNDAMENTALS

FEEL LIKE SOMETHING RICH AND CREAMY?

Every second of life your body is under constant destruction and reconstruction. This is the normal state of being alive and it provides great opportunities to rebuild, however late in the game one decides to start.

Some tissues replace themselves rapidly. The platelets for example, are cells that you now have in your blood that did

125

not exist two weeks ago. Billions and billions of them, thousands in each drop of blood. They turn over totally every two weeks. The red cells that circulate with them did not exist four months ago. Billions and billions of them. Every tissue in the body is in a similar state of dismantling and reconstruction. As new building blocks from the food in your diet are incorporated into the system, they gradually displace the ones from the old ways that are being recycled.

This brings us to one of the major roles of fat in life, mainly to create flexibility of all cell walls, membranes and cell wrappings. The basic construction unit of all tissues in the body is the cell, a tiny ball or box with walls that are made of fat. Cell walls are layered membranes: a layer of protein on the outside, a layer of protein on the inside and layers of fat in between. But the layers of fat in all membranes are perpendicular to the plane of the membrane. So imagine a sardine sandwich with the sardines in the center representing the fat molecules. The slice of bread on the top half is the outside layer, then the perpendicular sardines, with noses touching the top side of the bread and tails touching the bottom side and layer. The sandwich is greatly thickened by the billions and billions of sardines representing the billions and billions of fat molecules that make up membrane. This arrangement enables molecules crossing membranes to make their way through by simply separating spaces between the molecules of fat.

Next you must understand that these sardines are alive and thrashing around in the membrane. It is a very turbulent system; the sardines are flipping from position to position always, however, maintaining their noses in contact with the outer layer and their tails in contact with the inner layer. In the process, great holes come and go, exchanges are made and replacements can be introduced. That's the way that a dietary change of fat eventually produces a change in the cells of the tissues of the body.

"MOST INDIVIDUALS THINK OF FAT AS SOLID, BUT IN THE BODY IT'S ALL LIQUID AND DEPENDING ON ITS BASIC CONSTRUCTION (SATURATED OR UNSATURATED) IT IS RELATIVELY STIFF OR RELATIVELY FLEXIBLE."

This is a new concept to grasp. Most individuals think of fat as solid, but in the body it's all liquid and depending on its basic construction (saturated or unsaturated) it is relatively stiff or relatively flexible. As a structural component of cell walls and membranes, the type and amount of fat we eat contributes to health and disease, the disease of today...the cancers and the heart attacks; as well as a lot of aches and pains.

127

Much of today's aching and paining is the result of the nature of membranes in the platelets that are constructed with the wrong kinds of fats. We must begin to understand fats as tissue components and construction components in the body which brings us to newer thinking on unsaturated fats. The more flexible the fats and oils you have in the membranes and tissues of your body, the more comfortable and easier it will be for all your tissues to move within themselves and around themselves; the more comfortably and easily will you move in the environment; the more flexible your movement of joints and tendons and ligiments.

A platelet's job is two-fold: To protect the breaks in the wall of the vascular tree and to prevent infection. It does these two things when it goes to pieces. It releases clotting agents that seal up the hole and it releases inflammatory agents that begin to protect against any invading bacteria that may have come in through the hole. By shatterproofing one's platelets (by making them very flexible so that they don't go to pieces very readily) one can minimize one's risk of forming a clot inside the blood (as in heart attacks and strokes and phlebitis), and one can reduce one's spontaneous level of aches and pains (as in arthritis, rheumatism and lumbago).

128

" THE THINGS WE'RE EATING THESE DAYS ARE NOT MAKING US WHAT WE WANT TO BE."

O n the national scene fat is in the fire. Back in 1986 full page newspaper ads on the hazards of tropical oils were paid for by one outraged postcoronary businessman. With no other motivation than trying to clean up the nation's diet, he began a one-man crusade. But other businessmen have other motivations. Enter the soybean processors.

An oil war erupted over fats and health, as feuding factions accused rival oils with responsibility for compromising the nation's health. In September of 1987 tempers in the Pacific ran so high that riot police had to be called out to protect the U.S. Embassy in Malaysia's capital city. Protesters opposed to tropical oil bad-mouthing were threatening the building and its staff. A month later, peace talks led to palm oil producers promising to quit the U.S. market if soy oil producers would quit talking about cholesterol.

Palm oil and coconut oil consist of 50% saturated fats. This can raise cholesterol in the bloodstream and increase the risk of a heart attack. Soy oil, on the other hand, the risk of a heart attack. Soy oil, on the other hand, contains only 15% saturated fat (although when used as margarine it must be partially hydrogenated which takes soy's saturated fat levels to 25%).

The soy oilers are upset that on food packages their product gets equal billing with coconut oil and palm oil, and in 1990 they were lobbying Congress to change this food labeling. For all the hoopla, the charges and countercharges, the simple truth, on both sides, is that the things we're eating these days are not making us what we want to be. Fats and oils from all producers and all sources are excessive. They contribute to 50% of the day's calories, and good evidence shows them to be tightly associated with today's diseases and disabilities.

Americans consume 80 million doses of pain killer a day, generally for headaches or joint and muscle pains, treating the complaints that result from inflammation. At a medical meeting in New York in 1986, a meeting devoted to managing inflammation, doctors discussed not only new forms of pain killers, but new dietary approaches to the problem as well. They took a fresh look at the role of fats and oils in provoking pain and the role of fish oils in mitigating it.

Inflammation is a basic reaction to any noxious event. It starts with the release of a compound into the tissues, a compound called arachidonic acid. Dietary fats and oils provide the raw material for building arachidonic acid. Arachidonic acid is a fatty molecule that's present in most cells of the body. The American diet provides 10 times the amount we need, and as the New York meeting showed, these excess intakes contribute to arachidonic acid excess that promotes aches and pains.

Excessive intakes of fats and oils, polyunsaturated fats included, assure high tissue levels of arachidonic acid. Their easy and voluminous release at sites of irritation produce the aches and pains that pain killers suppress. Cutting back on polyunsaturated and saturated fat intakes, by more than 50%, often reduces the aches and pains and the need for any pain killers at all. But beyond the simple strategy of cutting back, adding certain special oils to the diet can produce a further reduction in aches and pains as the scientists discovered. Enter fish oils.

Researchers, reporting at the meeting, found that the omega-3 oils of ocean fish produce a significant reduction in pain in at least a third of patients suffering such chronic pain conditions as arthritis, headaches and phlebitis. Others at the Medical School in Albany, New York, have confirmed something that patients with arthritis have known for years: Certain foods have an influence on their symptoms. Cutting fats, the doctors found, reduces the pain, especially the pain of active rheumatoid arthritis.

131

> *"...THE FATS AND OILS WE EAT ENTER OUR BLOODSTREAMS TO JOIN AN ENORMOUS FLOATING SUPPLY OF TISSUE BUILDING MATERIALS AND MOLECULES."*

T he New York investigators did a classical controlled study, and they limited the test fats to saturated fats. That's the kind in meat and dairy products but not the kind that are in fish or corn oil. It was a double blind study, meaning that neither clinician nor patient knew which diet had the saturated fat. Nearly 40 patients were in the study and all had active rheumatoid arthritis. After 12 weeks the results revealed a clear, if modest, difference in the two groups. On the low saturated fat diet there was less morning stiffness, less pain and tenderness. Most of the improvement, however, did not become evident until the third month of the study. And when the benefited patients returned to their usual diets they only deteriorated after a delay of several weeks to the same level of discomfort and disability as before. Remember those tissue turnover paragraphs at the beginning of this chapter?

Long-term intakes of fish oil supplements can help reconstruct the body's tissues by replacing the onboard

132

saturated fats. They produce less of an inflammatory response to everyday injury. The fats and oils we eat enter the bloodstream to join the floating supply of building materials. When the nature of the fat in the cell membrane wall sandwich is changed to incorporate more omega-3 marine oil, the resulting cells are more flexible. As circulating platelets they become more shatter-proof and less aggravating, less stiff and sticky.

SELF CARE IS THE ONLY
HEALTH INSURANCE

FITNESS FEEDINGS

CLEAN GRAIN WHEATCAKES

1-1/3 cups whole wheat flour
2 tsp baking powder
1 egg, slightly beaten
1-1/3 cups milk
1 T brown sugar, packed
1 T oil

Grease griddle (see note). Heat the griddle while mixing the batter. The griddle is hot enough when drops of water sprinkled on it will bounce. Mix flour and baking powder. Beat egg, milk, sugar and oil together. Add liquid mixture to flour mixture. Stir only until flour is moistened. The batter will be slightly lumpy. For each pancake, pour about 1/4 cup batter onto the hot griddle. Cook until covered with bubbles and the edges are slightly dry. Turn and brown the other side.

NOTE: It is generally unnecessary to grease a well-seasoned griddle or one with a non-stick surface.

COACH'S CORNER

CLEAN SHOPPING TRICKS

A key part in learning to eat healthfully is clean shopping, and being organized is a must. If possible, plan for the week ahead and prepare a list of ingredients you'll need to buy, allowing for those things you already have. This cuts down on your tendency to buy impulse foods.

Try to shop on a full stomach and preferably alone. This allows you to get in and out of the store quickly and to stick to The Plan.

Once in the store remember that 50% of purchased food has been shown to be bought on impulse, and that's the kind you don't need. Retailers increase impulse buying by displaying the most expensive and most processed foods at eye level. Such foods almost always highly processed contain excessive amounts of fat, salt or sugar.

Rather than browse up and down the aisles, shop the walls, the store's outer edges. There you'll find fruits, vegetables, dairy products, breads, chicken, and fish. The few products you must shop the aisles for, are usually located out of eye level on bottom shelves. You'll have to shop for them.

7 | FOOD SENSITIVITY FUNDAMENTALS

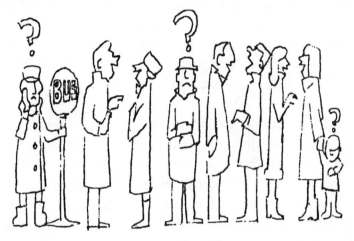

COULD IT BE SOMETHING YOU ATE?

J ust how many of us are allergic or sensitive to food is uncertain, but it's not a small number. If minor reactions like skin itching, headache, nasal stuffiness and abdominal bloating are included, then probably one in four Americans is affected. And that's millions of us suffering needlessly.

137

Food reactions and sensitivities express themselves in three ways. There are the potential perturbations of the metabolic system as shown by reactive hypoglycemia. There are digestive expressions like bloating, tenderness, nausea constipation and diarrhea; and there are allergic expressions. All have the potential to affect mood and behavior, within minutes, hours, and even days. Watchful wariness is the only approach that makes sense until the details of an emerging problem are defined.

In our lifetime we've changed not only our food ways, but our food composition, and both continue to evolve. We eat fewer calories than our parents and far fewer than our grandparents. Fast foods, snack foods, vended foods, frozen foods, and convenience foods make frequent contacts a simple and everyday practice. We are a nation of nibblers and grazers, and the pasture for all this is everywhere. Foods for that pasture must be carefully conditioned, ever-fresh and ever-ready, meaning that many chemical modifications are required as precautions against rancidity and deterioration. Some of these modifications express themselves in our reactions to the food once consumed.

The most effective way to discover whether or not certain foods are making you tired or depressed or feel funny is to eliminate them from your diet for a couple of weeks and then challenge yourself with several servings of them for each of two consecutive days. Watch for an effect over the following few days. Foods that are commonly associated with sensitivity reactions such as shaking, trembling, congestion, fatigue and depression are dairy products, wheat products, corn products, eggs and cane sugar.

That food could be associated with non-life threatening, almost chronic complaints is only slowly being accepted by physicians. Take for example, food and arthritis. Many patients say there's a relationship. Many arthritis doctors deny it. Risking the professional disapproval of fellow physicians for practicing "fringe medicine" several British arthritis specialists reported in 1985 an experiment with diet and rheumatoid arthritis. In a very scientific manner they observed the effect of food on their patients' joint pains and on their sense of well-being. They concluded that modifying the diet helped the arthritis sufferers.

> *"THE STUDY DEMONSTRATED THAT FOOD HAS A SIGNIFICANT INFLUENCE ON MORNING STIFFNESS, PAINFUL JOINTS AND MUSCLE STRENGTH."*

Because the role of food in rheumatoid arthritis and most other kinds of arthritis remains controversial, a double blind experimental design had been undertaken. This meant that neither doctor nor patient knew which was in the test group and which in the control. All patients went on a two-week "wash out" period before the study began. Medication was withdrawn and they ate a diet generally recognized to be associated with few allergic symptoms -- rice, lamb, and selected fruits and vegetables; after which they were allocated in a random way to either food capsule challenge for a week or dummy food capsule challenge. Then the procedure was reversed.

The study demonstrated that food has a significant influence on morning stiffness, painful joints and muscle strength. About 15% of the arthritis sufferers improved dramatically and about 15% did not benefit at all. The remaining 70% showed varying degrees of benefit. The aggravating foods were those commonly found to produce food sensitivities: dairy products, wheat, corn, citrus, coffee and chocolate. Not every food upset every patient. There were highly individualized responses.

In speculating on the use of this information to manage rheumatoid arthritis the researchers were cautious: Some patients with rheumatoid arthritis can be expected to benefit, but not everyone. Future research should develop screens for individual patients likely to experience benefit and then focus on determining why the foods are aggravating.

This report was just one in a continuing series of scientific evaluations of the role of dietary manipulation in treating many common complaints. Given today's concerns about the side effects and costs of many new drugs, a look at diet therapy or at least the identification of aggravating diet items not only makes economic sense, but is becoming scientifically respectable.

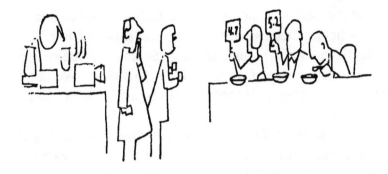

T he more we modify food, and the more we engineer it, the greater our likelihood of trouble, the greater our likelihood of creating or introducing unusual molecules to which some of us may become sensitive. Each of us is highly individual. Just as our fingertips are unique in their imprints, so is much of our chemistry. For this reason the problems of food sensitivity must be faced in the clinic and not the laboratory. On the self-help front, don't ignore food that works poorly on you whatever unaffected friends might think or say. Living defensively these days involves a little eccentricity. If you are in any way disconcerted after any food or drink, avoid it. Period.

However good it tastes, if it bites you, stop setting yourself up. One recent case concerned a patient with repeated allergic reactions to the flavor-enhancer monosodium glutamate. It's not a rare reaction. What was unusual about the case was the delay. He had no symptoms until 18-24 hours after exposure. The mechanism of this long delay is unknown but not uncommon, and it's one reason for so many missed food sensitivity diagnoses. We don't realize that yesterday's food can still be affecting us today.

Research done on 43 children with recurrent complaints of itching and hives revealed that 24 of them were reacting to common food additives. The mechanisms of their intolerance did not depend on the immune response because they did not react to classic skin tests. It was only when challenged double-blind by capsules that the hives occurred, and the mechanism of this response is not known. The additives responsible were common dyes and preservatives. So reactions to foods can take place a day later, and they need not show up in the classic allergy test-- a confusing states of affairs.

To compound the problem, we eat a diet of increasing chemical complexity. For reasons of appearance, taste, convenience, texture, shelf-life and cost, it's the food we want   the way we want it although it requires much chemical manipulation.   While the chemicals used are submitted to rigorous animal and laboratory tests before clearance for human use, clinical concerns are mounting over what is really a large-scale human feeding experiment that has been under way for several decades on the populations of industrialized countries.

Today's foods contain a growing concentration of novel molecules, including the additives just mentioned as well as new molecules created in food by processing.   The temperatures and pressures employed in commercial processing are enormous.   To remove the corn taste and odor from corn oil for example, the high temperature and pressure produce unusual fats in the final product.   The fats are known as trans-fatty acids.   They do not exist in nature and cannot be utilized in the normal way when studied in biological systems. Fed to test animals in large amounts, they give the animals sick brains.

"TODAY'S FOODS CONTAIN A GROWING CONCENTRATION OF NOVEL MOLECULES, CREATED IN FOOD BY PROCESSING."

A 1983 report on levels of trans-fatty acids in the American diet revealed that we eat one to two teaspoons of them a day. This is an intake that has not changed over the past two decades and a body burden that does not seem to be hurting us. But trans-fatty acids, food dyes and food preservatives are just three examples of novelty nutrients continuing to enter our diet. There are unusual proteins in soy protein products which come from the high temperatures and pressure manipulation of soy beans. There is also a growing number of wetting agents, blenders and extenders and other elements of food technology expertise.

Alone or in combination, they can surface as clinical problems--perhaps as rashes or wheezing that make allergic associations easily recognizable, perhaps as other disorders that are even more common. What about fatigue and depression? It's so general a complaint these days that psychiatrists are searching for "agent blue" to account for their case loads of depressed patients. Could one element in the challenge be strange ingredients in their patients' diets? Blood sugar blues are not the only association of food and mood but they are real too.

People who are sensitive to sugar may be reacting to its contained plant protein allergens. They might be sensitive to the protein of grass pollen in cane sugar for example, but not to the plant proteins of beet sugar, honey or maple sugar. Hypoglycemia is a sugar reaction

144

that is very common and has nothing to do with allergy. It is the result of an over sensitive sugar digestion and disposal mechanism as in the case of the patient described below.

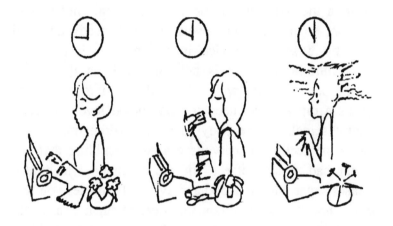

About 10 o'clock most mornings, the patient had "sinking spells"; attacks of tiredness, nervousness and trembling. At such times, she also felt hungry, had something to eat and felt better. Friends said it sounded like low blood sugar. The doctor ordered tests which showed a low blood sugar, and everyone was pleased. Her friends recommended a high protein diet but the doctor was more interested in a greater change in her ways.

145

On a typical day, she had a sweet roll for breakfast or the kids' leftover cereal, plus some fruit juice and a couple of cups of coffee. Mid-mornings, for the sinking spells, she took a cookie and coffee. Such a diet is rich in carbohydrates and caffeine, and often leads to blood sugar dips.

Sugar in the blood is vital to life. The brain needs it to function, so blood sugar levels are held steady day and night by a sensing device in the brain; just as the temperature in a house is held steady by a thermostat sensing device on the wall. When the sugar "thermostat" signals a dip and the need to raise blood levels it sends electric signals to the body to release adrenalin.   This causes the feeling of nervousness and trembling that our patient had, a side effect of the adrenalin which also releases sugar into the blood and eventually makes you feel better; not as quickly of course, as eating sugar or a snack, but as effectively. The caffeine in her coffee also acted like adrenalin.   It didn't raise her blood sugar, but it did heighten her feelings of nervousness and trembling.

Many of today's hypoglycemia victims eat a light carbohydrate breakfast and drink coffee. After such a breakfast, the blood sugar rises sharply for an hour or two then just as sharply falls and triggers symptoms. Our patient's spells were the result of a dip in her blood sugar and a squirt of adrenalin on top of caffeine. Prevention of the problem works best if carbohydrate and caffeine are both reduced; and this is the usual management. It is sometimes described incorrectly as a high-protein diet, an incomplete prescription. The sugars that trigger symptoms can be replaced by complex carbohydrates such as whole grain oatmeal sugars with their fiber, -or the orange rather than the orange juice.

By focusing only on food however, we ignore the role of physical inactivity in this syndrome of the blood sugar blahs. Muscles can play an important part in treating the condition. Physical activity is as important as food in smoothing out our patient's kind of low blood sugar. Look for example, at kids.

"BY FOCUSING ONLY ON FOOD, HOWEVER, WE IGNORE THE ROLE OF PHYSICAL INACTIVITY IN THIS SYNDROME OF THE BLOOD SUGAR BLAHS."

When kids in school get restless, it's usually from a normal, 10 AM, slight degree of hypoglycemia, so we declare recess and send them outside for 15 minutes of romping in the playground. It restores their blood sugars to normal and they return to class relaxed and refreshed. Exercise does this by restoring balance, by adjustments that go well

147

beyond the oversimplified notion of spike and dip, of sugar in and sugar out. For mothers at home or on the job, household or office chores these days are seldom energy-demanding and don't provide any blood sugar balancing benefits. The next time you get that mid-morning dip, don't eat, but declare recess and take a brisk walk (or put on some music and dance a bit). It'll sweeten up the rest of your morning, naturally.

EAT AS LITTLE AS POSSIBLE ON FAITH

COACH'S CORNER

FUNNY REACTIONS TO FOOD

Despite the distance we've come in our understanding of food and health, we have only an incomplete
appreciation regarding relationships between food
and mood, food and performance, food and behavior.

Day-to-day, many individuals experience chronic
low grade adverse reactions to food such as recurring
headaches, gut aches, fatigue, or episodes of
unexplained agitation or depression. These and other
food-related reactions often go unrecognized.

There are two broad categories of adverse reactions
to food. One is acute, with symptoms tightly tied to
food exposure time-wise, so the relationship is easily
recognized. Collapsing or wheezing after eating
something is a common example.

In the second type of reaction, the relationship of
symptoms to food is less obvious. Symptoms may
develop a day or two after the food encounter,
producing recurring headaches, joint pains, fatigue
and even depression. Binge eating is common and
can contribute to a weight problem in susceptible individuals.

PART THREE

IT'S ALL ABOUT NUMBERS

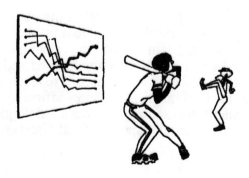

IS IT IMPORTANT TO SET GOALS ?

...ONLY IF YOU CARE WHERE YOU'RE GOING.

S tudies of human behavior confirm in many ways that goal-setting optimizes outcomes. New Year's resolutions are perhaps the most obvious examples of points in the year when we take inventory and plot a few new strategies for the future. Vague objectives such as "being the best" or "giving my all" are too diffuse to produce any measurable improvement.

Goals that work are well defined. Indeed they are often single issue items like losing 10 pounds or walking for 15 minutes a day. Rewards for achieving these goals should be equally well defined: perhaps a trip, or clothes or jewelry or a book or gadget.

Be reasonable. Setting sights too high is discouraging. The best goals are within reach with a reasonable amount of effort. By avoiding frustration the emotional energy needed to hold one's course remains focused and leads to success. Perfection should not be needed to reach any goal. Perfection is for God, as many cultures affirm in different ways. Reasonable goal setting involves a little organization and planning plus a certain amount of self discipline.

STEP 1: **Define your goal in hard terms.**

Whether it's food habits, fitness habits or   recreation activities. **Be specific.**

STEP 2: **Identify problem elements.**

What might interfere?   Relatives?   Associates? Unpredictable assignments? Competing interests? Limits of time or money? **Plan ahead.**

STEP 3: **Set a time frame.**

Perhaps it's one daily serving of fresh fruit, or green vegetables. Perhaps its a brief daily walk.   Perhaps it's getting professional help. **Starting today.**

STEP 4: **Make a commitment.**

Be serious. Be dedicated. Be tough.   Say "no" a few times. Write your new activity down then post it up somewhere. **Find the time .**

STEP 5: **Keep a record.**

Measure progress. Life is a process and keeping score not only reminds you of progress but allows for adjusting and reevaluating. **Keep score.**

TAKING INVENTORY
using the ScoreCard and ScoreBoard

Anyone looking for full performance and energetic
longevity must start:

* looking at some health-promoting habits.
* looking at some health-undermining habits.
* following some health indicators such as
the resting heart rate
the body weight
the blood pressure
and
the blood cholesterol

Having taken inventory or established a baseline, the next
step toward better health or better prospects is to make
some changes and track those changes over the months,
keeping track of them and their effect on the wellness
numbers.

Let's look again at Martin K ...

154

MARTIN K: A Case Study In Goal Setting

The health concern that brought him to my office and led to a re-examination of his lifestyle was a simple enough event, a breathless episode, but it led eventually to several major losses and some very gratifying gains.

It all began when he encountered an important associate waiting for an elevator in the lobby of their building. Martin suggested they climb the three flights to their floor and discuss some confidential new business as they went. He began to set out his department's position on the issue only to have his breath leave him before reaching the second floor .

He tried to dismiss it, joking about his weight (although he didn't have a visible problem) with a comment about getting into shape one-of-these-days. His wife, however, was not so easily mollified when he told her the story that evening. She sensed his concern and felt a tiny chill of alarm herself. In fact, it was she who made the appointment for him to come in for a check-up. As men will, his first words to me gave her full credit/blame. "My wife sent me in," he explained.

During the preliminary evaluation, his problems were not long in surfacing, problems now known as health risk factors, problems called abnormal findings, problems that roadmap a path to major mischief ahead.

155

At 183 pounds, Martin K was 25 pounds heavier than he'd been in his twenties. His heart sounded strong and steady and his EKG showed no damage. But his resting rate of 84 beats per minute, his blood pressure of 135/80 and his cholesterol of 232 were not reassuring. All contributed to the picture of a sedentary lifestyle and a fatty foodstyle, setting the stage for a heart attack or stroke. During a treadmill stress test he called a halt to proceedings after only 8 minutes because of breathlessness.

His other findings were not so disturbing. His blood sugar was 80, and the rest of his chemistries and counts were also normal.

As you'll recall from the earlier section, when he sat down to the scorecards to take inventory of his habits, good and bad, he arrived at a Total Score that was less than impressive. He now entered all his numbers and symbols in the first column of the ScoreBoard as shown on the opposite page.

The next step was to determine how to go about improving on them.Martin was something of an efficiency expert. He decided to introduce some changes into his well-established routines, to continue to go with the daily flow but where possible replace a few destructive elements in his day with constructive ones.

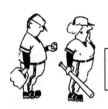

WINNING

MARTIN K

S GAME

YOUR PRESEASON
ScoreBoard™

THE   **ROOKIES**

YOUR FIRST AT-BATS IN THE GAME

SCORE SCALE	YOUR SCORE TODAY	AFTER ONE WEEK	AFTER TWO WEEKS	AFTER THREE WEEKS	AFTER FOUR WEEKS	SYMBOLS
300						**CHOLESTROL**
260						©
240	© 232					Fasting blood cholesterol well under 200 is ideal
210						
						BODYWEIGHT
200						ⓦ
190						Enter today's weight
	ⓦ 183					**BLD. PRESSR**
180						ⓟ
170						Systolic blood pressure under 120 mm Hg is ideal
160						**TOTAL SCORE**
150						ⓣ
140						The global view of your progress. Above 200 ideal.
	ⓟ 135					**BLOOD SUGR**
130						ⓢ
120	ⓣ 120					Fasting blood sugar under 90 is ideal
110						**HEART RATE**
100						ⓗ
90						A resting heart rate under 60 beats per minute is ideal
80	ⓗ 84					**NEXT MONTH:** (USING SYMBOLS) ENTER TODAY'S SCORE IN SCORE SCALE COLUMN OF SEASON'S PLAY ScoreCard
70						
60						
50						

IT'S ALL ABOUT NUMBERS. GET TO KNOW THE WELLNESS RANGE.

His blood sugar, (S) 80, was normal, so he felt he could safely ignore that. But his cholesterol (C) was alarming and he determined to give immediate attention to correcting the fat and fiber imbalance in his diet.

For breakfast, the bacon and eggs would be replaced by grapefruit, oatmeal and maple syrup. It was so simple, he began to prepare his own before leaving for work.

For lunch, he would brown bag it: an apple, pear or peach to go with a whole wheat pita pocket sandwich of tomatoes, cucumber or tuna. This replaced the executive burger and pickles. His wife, wholly supportive, prepared and refrigerated lunch the night before.

Martin also knew that measures to improve his physical fitness would have to be embedded in his daily routine as well. Evenings he usually arrived home to sit before television and have pre-dinner drinks (a fifth of scotch a week). These were replaced with sparkling water or wine, and he would retire a half hour earlier to get up to go out into the neighborhood before work. Donning togs appropriate to the season, he sensibly started a walking program.

In all, it was a significant change in lifestyle habit patterns, and as can be seen on the next page, a downward trend emerged associated with the sharp upward trend of Martin's most telling number, his Total Score, (T).

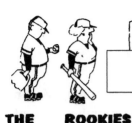

WINNING S GAME

MARTIN K

YOUR PRESEASON ScoreBoard™

THE   ROOKIES

YOUR FIRST AT-BATS IN THE GAME

SCORE SCALE	YOUR SCORE TODAY	AFTER ONE WEEK	AFTER TWO WEEKS	AFTER THREE WEEKS	AFTER FOUR WEEKS	SYMBOLS
300						**CHOLESTROL** © Fasting blood cholesterol well under 200 is ideal
260						
240	© 232					
210					© 210	**BODYWEIGHT** ⓦ Enter today's weight
200						
190					ⓣ 190	**BLD. PRESSR** ⓟ Systolic blood pressure under 120 mm Hg is ideal
180	ⓦ 183					
170		ⓦ	ⓦ	ⓦ	ⓦ 170	
160						**TOTAL SCORE** ⓣ The global view of your progress. Above 200 ideal.
150						
140						
130	ⓟ 135					**BLOOD SUGR** ⓢ Fasting blood sugar under 90 is ideal
120	ⓣ 120				ⓟ 125	
110						**HEART RATE** ⓗ A resting heart rate under 60 beats per minute is ideal
100						
90						
80	ⓗ 84	ⓗ	ⓗ	ⓗ		**NEXT MONTH:** (USING SYMBOLS) ENTER TODAY'S SCORE IN SCORE SCALE COLUMN OF SEASON'S PLAY ScoreCard
70					ⓗ 70	
60						
50						

IT'S ALL ABOUT NUMBERS. GET TO KNOW THE WELLNESS RANGE.

MARTIN K's WINNING SEASON

Encouraged by the success of his try-out month, Martin continued his performance over a full six month season of play. Look at his graph on the next page.

Things went well during the first few months, but in the fifth month when he combined a business convention with a week of vacation in Las Vegas, he suffered a setback, not a major setback, and one from which he quickly recovered.

Looking at some of his individual issues over the first season, Martin's cholesterol responded nicely to his change in diet, starting at 232 and reaching 200 at the end. His starting weight of 183 was not ideal (160) but after 6 months was closer to target and he was pleased to be able to carry on a conversation while climbing stairs once again. Notice how his fitness program (just brisk walking) lowered the resting heart rate (H) from a starting rate of 84 beats a minute to a slow and efficient rate of 54. That's a weight-controlling, breath-enhancing outcome.

Martin's fifth month departure from form when he and his wife had the western holiday, did no lasting damage as you can see. It was just a hiccup on the chart. Once back into his health promoting new routine, working with the grain of his tissues rather than with medications, his new ways continued to make his internal environment even healthier.

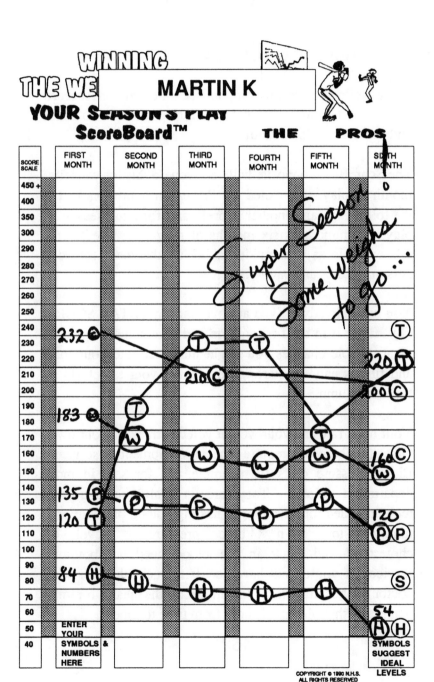

TRACKING YOUR OWN PROGRESS

In the wellness game, keeping an accurate and honest score is as important as in any game, offering triumphs to savor and setbacks to learn from.

The ScoreBoard opposite will help you do this for your first month of play. It's called the Preseason ScoreBoard. On the following page another ScoreBoard, for a full season of play, accommodates six months of progress. Use Martin K's example as your guide, taking all the space for your personal notes and cautions.

You have already arrived at your starting TOTAL SCORE (T). Enter it in the first column and give some thought to what do-able changes you might introduce into your food and fitness patterns starting now. Enter your target (T) in the last column.

Your heart rate and your weight you can track on your own. Other numbers will require special equipment or services. Blood pressure cuffs for example, are for sale in most department stores. They are generally reliable and recommended for anyone who has high blood pressure or a family history of high blood pressure. Levels of cholesterol and sugar in the blood need a laboratory service. If you do not have access to such (through your doctor or hospital) take advantage of the health-o-ramas that many shopping malls hold from time to time.

162

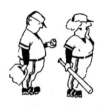

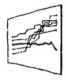

WINNING
THE WELLNESS GAME

YOUR PRESEASON
ScoreBoard™

THE   ROOKIES

YOUR FIRST AT-BATS IN THE GAME

SCORE SCALE	YOUR SCORE TODAY	AFTER ONE WEEK	AFTER TWO WEEKS	AFTER THREE WEEKS	AFTER FOUR WEEKS	SYMBOLS
300						
260						**CHOLESTROL** © Fasting blood cholesterol well under 200 is ideal
240						
210						
200						**BODYWEIGHT** Ⓦ Enter today's weight
190						
180						**BLD. PRESSR** Ⓟ Systolic blood pressure under 120 mm Hg is ideal
170						
160						**TOTAL SCORE** Ⓣ The global view of your progress. Above 200 ideal.
150						
140						
130						**BLOOD SUGR** Ⓢ Fasting blood sugar under 90 is ideal
120						
110						**HEART RATE** Ⓗ A resting heart rate under 60 beats per minute is ideal
100						
90						
80						**NEXT MONTH:** (USING SYMBOLS) ENTER TODAY'S SCORE
70						
60						IN SCORE SCALE COLUMN OF
50						SEASON'S PLAY ScoreCard

IT'S ALL ABOUT NUMBERS. GET TO KNOW THE WELLNESS RANGE.

YOUR SEASON'S PLAY, AND BEYOND

Changing habits and numbers in any meaningful way takes time, and the benefits that follow take time to express themselves. Be patient. You are reversing patterns that took a lifetime to get to where they are.

Persistence will gradually normalize most of the numbers on the opposite page. Payoffs will not be dramatic but they will be *enduring* and usually free from side effects.

Natural processes will produce a replacement and repair from a simple change in your diet. It's never too late to benefit, but the older you are and the more tentative, the slower and less complete will be the benefits. Individuals in their middle years cannot expect decades of faulty tissue construction from a faulty diet to be repaired in weeks. It takes months and years, but take place it does. So get started.

WINNING THE WELLNESS GAME
YOUR SEASON'S PLAY
ScoreBoard™

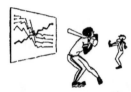

THE   PROS

SCORE SCALE	FIRST MONTH	SECOND MONTH	THIRD MONTH	FOURTH MONTH	FIFTH MONTH	SIXTH MONTH
450 +						
400						
350						
300						
290						
280						
270						
260						
250						
240						Ⓣ
230						
220						
210						
200						
190						
180						
170						
160						Ⓒ
150						
140						
130						
120						
110						Ⓟ
100						
90						
80						Ⓢ
70						
60						
50	ENTER YOUR					Ⓗ
40	SYMBOLS & NUMBERS HERE					SYMBOLS SUGGEST IDEAL LEVELS

PART FOUR

SHORT CUTS TO THE MAJORS

A CAUTIONARY NOTE REGARDING THESE INSIGHT OUTLINES

"SHAKE WELL BEFORE USING"

This traditional label on bottled medicine applies equally to bottled information. Shake the information in this section up with your own experience and with past medical advice. Do not undertake any action options outlined in this section before discussing them and showing them to your personal physician. Ask if there is any conflict with your current health care program, medications, or past susceptibilities. Follow the personal advice you get, not your own interpretation of the information contained in this section.

The documented benefits of habit change are long-term and cannot be expected short term. They are gradual, continuing and measurable benefits that come from gradual, continuing and measurable change.

But we are impatient creatures, wanting some evident return on investment now, within days rather than months, weeks rather than seasons. So the following quick start guides were developed to help you take those first tentative steps and overcome inertia.

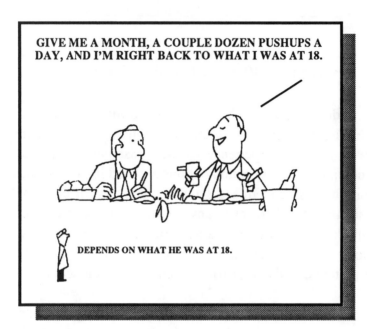

FOOD SUPPLEMENT ACTION STEPS

DAILY VITAMINS AND MINERALS

...AN OVERVIEW

Although attitudes are changing, physicians in general still disapprove of taking food supplements such as vitamins and minerals. "Get all your nutrient needs from the food you eat," they say. But there are serious problems with this advice, based as it is on the assumption that the average American adult eats at least 1800 calories a day, and on other assumptions about the source of those calories. For example: Many weight conscious women eat fewer than 1400 calories a day, food intakes that cannot provide adequate vitamins and minerals.

Beyond this simple consideration of getting adequate amounts of trace nutrients to prevent deficiency, a great deal of scientific evidence has accumulated which indicates that large doses of isolated vitamins, or minerals and certain food constituents (doses beyond those needed to prevent deficiency but not large enough to cause illness) have specific health promoting benefits. They are highlighted on the following pages.

171

ASCORBATE. Vitamin C is an anti-oxidant and controlled studies on animals given the human equivalent of 3 grams a day, have demonstrated increased longevity of rabbits and mice by 25% and increased resistance to infections.

Megadose Risks: *Generally viewed as nontoxic, but very high doses such as 5 to 10 grams a day have caused gastritis (stomach upset) and kidney stones (overproduction of calcium oxalate) from breakdown products of vitamin C.*

BETA CAROTENE: More than 50 studies have associated the consumption of carotene with a reduced risk of cancer. A reversal of precancerous cells from the lung, mouth and cervix has also been shown.

Megadose Risks: *Within the body it is stored in all tissues so that taking large amounts can lead to orange skin discoloration best seen in palms and soles.*

CALCIUM: For preventing osteoporosis, doses of 1 to 2 grams a day are a very good idea up to age 30 for women. Beyond age 30 calcium supplements are not nearly as well documented a benefit as daily fitness, estrogens for a decade after the menopause and fluoride; but still not a bad idea. Calcium also has nerve sedative properties, so supplements may be useful with magnesium in leg cramps and the anxiety of stress.

Megadose Risks: *Kidney stone formers may want to weigh the risks and benefits. Although some patients with high blood pressure experience a lowering with calcium supplements, a few show elevations. Calcium for blood pressure must be monitored.*

FIBER: A natural promoter of daily laxation whether from a food source or as an isolate. It reduces the risk of diverticulitis, appendicitis, colon cancer and (with certain fibers) even heart attacks.

Megadose Risks: *Usually cramps and diarrhea, but on occasion, intestinal obstruction can result from taking too much.*

FISH OIL: Poly-poly unsaturated fats of marine origin which eventually become incorporated into the cell walls of all tissues of the body. This produces a number of different beneficial effects: lowered blood fats, less sticky platelets, fewer allergic reactions and reduced inflammations such as: arthritis, phlebitis, or migraine.

Megadose Risks: *Longer bleeding time for cuts and bruises. Fish breath or skin rash if fish sensitive.*

FLUORIDE: An established calcium crystal stabilizer in teeth and bones. Presently added to most municipal water supplies for cavity control, but several studies have suggested a benefit in osteoporosis.

Megadose Risks: *Mottling of the teeth and mottling of the skeleton on X-rays. Chronic low back pain.*

FOLATE: Doses of 10 mg. a day have been shown to reverse to normal precancerous cells from cervix and lungs.

Megadose Risks: *Unknown, awaiting long-term studies.*

IRON: Doses in excess of 15 mg. a day should only be taken by individuals with iron deficiency anemia- usually women during their reproductive years.

Megadose Risks: *Excessive storage in susceptible individuals can lead to liver disease or disease of the pancreas.*

MAGNESIUM: Because of processing, it's a shrinking mineral in our diet. Has nerve sedative properties, so it may be useful with calcium in leg cramps and the anxiety of stress for a calming effect.

Megadose Risks: *Respiratory depression and low blood pressure.*

MULTIVITAMINS: A standard daily dose with iron for all adults makes good clinical sense. It should also contain B-12.

Megadose Risks: *Sensitivity states. Allergic reactions to starch binders.*

NIACIN: A B-vitamin for cholesterol control, but requires large doses and supervision.

Megadose Risks: *Facial flushing, headache, stomach upset.*

PHENYLALANINE: An amino acid precursor of brain chemicals called neurotransmitters. Supplements have mixed effects: sometimes calming, sometimes mood elevating.

Megadose Risks: *Unpredictable mood effects. Not for*

175

individuals with phenylketonuria.

PYRIDOXINE: Vitamin B-6 which calms nerve function and has been shown in several studies to have a benefit in the anxiety of stress, premenstrual tension and irritated peripheral nerves. It is a serotonin production promoter, especially when used with tryptophan.

Megadose Risks: *Nerve poisoning, numbness and tingling.*

SELENIUM: Many studies in laboratories show an anti-cancer effect. Promotes formation and activity of glutathione reductase, a ubiquitous tissue anti-oxidant.

Megadose Risks: *Congenital defects in offspring of laboratory animals.*

TOCOPHEROL: Vitamin E is an anti-oxidant with possible, but poorly documented anti-aging anti-cancer, anti-wrinkling benefits. Should work, but hard to document so far.

Megadose Risks: *Headache, hypertension, depression.*

176

TRYPTOPHAN: Amino acid precursor of catecholamine neurotransmitter serotonin. It has a calming, sleep-promoting anti-anxiety, anti-stress effect in most individuals.

Megadose Risks: *Drowsiness. Presently (1991) off the market because of a toxic contaminant which caused muscle disintegration and the deaths of at least 25 people. It was none the less a very effective sedative and calming agent for millions of people before a change in the manufacturing process lead to the hazardous product.*

TYROSINE: Amino acid precursor of catecholamine neurotransmitters. Taken for an energizing, anti-depressive effect on mood and behavior.

Megadose Risks: *Unpredictable mood effects.*

ZINC: Another essential mineral whose concentrations are slipping from our diet thanks to processing. Sketchy early studies suggest a role in minimizing the prostate enlargement that effects a third of men.

Megadose Risks: *Possible immune system compromise.*

FOOD SUPPLEMENTS CHECKLIST

TOWARD POORER HEALTH

☐ VITAMIN OR MINERAL "ENERGIZERS"

☐ PROTEIN SUPPLEMENTS

☐ UNPROVEN PERFORMANCE ENHANCERS

☐ OVER-THE-COUNTER "DIURETICS"

TOWARD BETTER HEALTH

☐ DAILY MULTI-VIT. (IF EATING LESS THAN 2000 CALS/DAY)

☐ DAILY MULTI-VIT. WITH IRON (WOMEN IN REPRODUCTIVE YRS.)

☐ DAILY CALCIUM 2-3 TUMS PER DAY (WOMEN)

☐ DAILY FIBER (PSYLLIUM FOR LAXATION, CHOLESTEROL)

☐ DAILY ANTIOXIDANT VIT. C 1000-3000 MG./ DAY

☐ DAILY ANTIOXIDANT VIT. E 400-800 IU / DAY

☐ DAILY ANTI-OXIDANT BETA CAROTENE 30MG / DAY

☐ DAILY ANTI-OXIDANT SELENIUM 50-100 MICROGRAMS / DAY

COACH'S CORNER

RE-THINKING SEASONINGS

America's favorite seasoning is salt, but there's a variety of alternative seasonings. Flavored vinegars, lemon juice, wine, sprinkle cheese, fresh or dried herbs, and spices are a few examples.

Start experimenting with fresh and dried herbs and spices. Use them sparingly and add them early on in food preparation so they can simmer with the other ingredients. Dried herbs are stronger, so use about 1/4 teaspoon of dried herbs for each teaspoon of fresh. After you become familiar with their flavors, increase the amount to compensate for the lack of salt.

Celery, spinach, and various greens such as beets, collards, chard, and kale tend to be higher in sodium than most vegetables. Simmer them along with your other ingredients. Their own sodium will help enhance the flavors of other ingredients. Bay leaves, fresh parsley, fresh dill, onions and peppercorns give stock and soups flavor without salt.

For built-in flavor, marinate poultry and fish for 24 hours with pepper, paprika, garlic and onion powder; or wine, lemon juice and the flavored vinegars. Experiment.

179

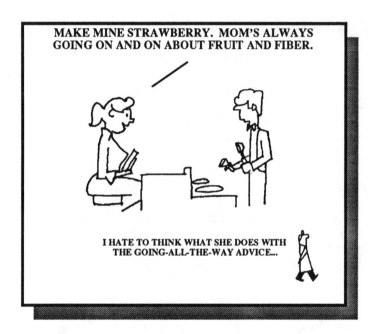

2 FOOD FIBER ACTION STEPS

WHERE'S FOOD FIBER?

...IN THIS DIET

Researchers in Alabama studied the eating effects of different diets on overweight and lean volunteers in an all-you-want-to-eat situation. The volunteers spent 2 weeks on 2 different diets -- one highly refined and tasty, the other whole food. They found that the volunteers got full satisfaction from as little as 1500 calories a day from whole food, but refined food only satisfied at levels of 3,000 calories a day.

Meal after meal, whether Clean or Dirty, the volunteers ate to satisfaction. Dirty breakfast options included: bacon, eggs, juice and buttered toast; fast foods and fried foods for lunch; and for dinner: roast and steak, hot dogs and hamburgers, buttered vegetables, whole milk, pie, cake, and ice cream. Eating to satisfaction required an average 3,000 calories each day, whether they were overweight or lean. Dirty dieting tastes good but isn't very filling.

181

During the Clean options week, breakfast provided: fresh fruits, hot cereals, skim milk, whole wheat toast and jam, tea or coffee; lunch provided: soups, salads and non-meat sandwiches; and for dinner they had: pasta, fish, chicken, rice, vegetables, whole wheat rolls and fruit. Eating all they wanted added up to 1,500 calories each day, whether they were overweight or lean. Clean eating tasted good and was twice as filling.

Clean eating helps keep the weight and blood pressure and sugar down; it helps keep the cholesterol down, and it helps prevent cancer...and there's more. A real bonus for people who like to eat, as the Alabama study showed, is that whole foods require 30% more eating time to put all those 1500 calories away. That's a third more time to eat half the calories. New math for the 90's for folks who like to eat.

A FIBERED FOODSTYLE CHECKLIST

TOWARD POORER HEALTH

- [ ] JUICED FRUIT OR CONCENTRATES
- [ ] PUREED VEGETABLES
- [ ] WHITE FLOUR PRODUCTS

TOWARD BETTER HEALTH

- [ ] VERY LEAN MEAT/CHICKEN/FISH ENTREE EMPHASIS
- [ ] DAILY FRUIT SEVERAL TIMES
- [ ] DAILY VEGETABLES HERBED AND SPICED
- [ ] DAILY PEAS, BEANS, LENTILS
- [ ] DAILY WHOLE GRAIN PRODUCTS
- [ ] DAILY WHOLE GRAIN CEREALS

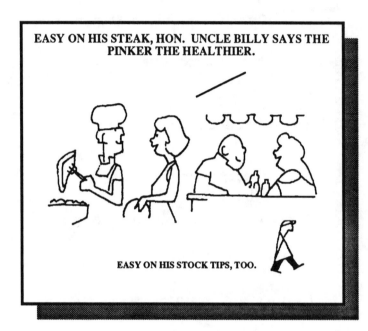

CHOLESTEROL ACTION STEPS

WHAT WILL CONTROL MY CHOLESTEROL?

...PERHAPS THE AA DIET OR THE AAA DIET

Heart attacks were rare 75 years ago and now they threaten to kill half of us. That it's largely a nutrition disease, thousands of studies have documented, and three basic food items have emerged as the responsible agents: fat, cholesterol and fiber. We must eat *less* fat, *less* cholesterol, and we must eat *more* fiber. These are the food principles underlying the two diets that follow.

As the research scrutinizes all types of fat, a few have been identified that are friendly to the heart, the unsaturates; and when the unsaturation involves the third carbon of the chain (Omega 3) the greatest benefits are achieved. These fats are commonly found in deep sea fish oils. They come from ocean plankton but land-based plant sources also occur, sources such as leafy green vegetables.

THE DOUBLE A DIET

By selecting from among the following foods, you'll be eating a diet that's low in cholesterol (< 200 mg.) and low in fat (< 25% of the calories). Portion sizes are not critical, unless you're watching calories.

SOME BREAKFAST SELECTIONS
Oatmeal with raisins, oranges, bran muffins, non-fat milk, coffee or tea. No butter, or margarine. English muffin or wheat toast w/jam or marmalade, yogurt w/walnuts, strawberries. Egg white omelette w/sauteed onions, tomatoes and green peppers, "Pam" fried or boiled potatoes, melon. Fresh fruit, shredded wheat, grape nuts.

SOME LUNCH SELECTIONS
Whole wheat pita pockets stuffed with sprouts or salad fixings no-oil dressing. Fruit plate or vegetable plate, sherbert, roll, jelly, coffee, tea. Herbed lentils w/rice, tossed salad w/no-oil dressing, bran muffin, non-fat milk. Whole wheat bread topped with tuna and salad made w/celery, onions and low-cal dressing. Non-creamed vegetable soup.

SOME DINNER SELECTIONS
Tossed salad w/no-oil dressing, poached halibut w/Parmesan cheese and lemon. Steamed whole grain brown rice, glazed pineapple carrots, fruit compote. Spinach lasagna, whole wheat bread, baked apple w/brown sugar. Chicken breasts in wine sauce, baked potato, ratatouille, Waldorf salad, coffee, tea. Pasta with tomato sauce topping, rice pudding, non-fat milk. Any lunch or breakfast selection.

SOME SNACK SELECTIONS
Hot air popcorn w/small amount of grated Parmesan cheese. Any fresh fruit. Oat bran muffins w/jam or marmalade and sugar-free chocolate. Non-fat yogurt topped with diced apples, walnuts, dates, raisins, fruit. Array of fresh vegetables w/non-fat yogurt dip. Grape Nuts in non-fat yogurt. Canned vegetables, hot or cold.

THE TRIPLE A DIET

This is a zero cholesterol diet. It provides the greatest possible cholesterol-lowering effect. It is a vegetarian diet including non-fat milk and egg whites. The selections are only guides.

SOME BREAKFAST SELECTIONS
Oatmeal w/raisins, oranges, bran muffins, non-fat milk, coffee, or tea. (No butter or margarine which, in a third of individuals   raises cholesterol.) Whole wheat English muffins w/corn oil margarine, jam, non-fat milk yogurt, egg white omelettes, fried potatoes with corn/safflower oil, whole wheat bread, baked beans and applesauce, pancakes (egg white) and syrup. Fresh fruit cup with toast, jelly.

SOME LUNCH SELECTIONS
Tomato and cucumber sandwich on whole wheat bread with seasoned corn/safflower oil dressing, vegetable soup, non-fat milk, pear, tea, ice water. Peanut butter and jelly sandwich. Non-fat cottage cheese (Breakstone) with crushed pineapple over baked potato, spinach salad with safflower oil dressing. Pasta salad with corn/safflower oil, bean soup, banana. Oat bran muffins w/marmalade.

SOME DINNER SELECTIONS
Bean enchiladas with tomato sauce, brown rice, tossed salad with corn/safflower oil dressing, fresh fruit medley, non-fat milk, tea. Herbed lentils with rice, broccoli-carrot stir-fry with corn/safflower oil. French bread with corn oil margarine, fruit compote. Vegetable soups. Bean and noodle casserole, roasted potatoes, julienne carrots and zucchini. Bean, pea or lentil soup. Brown rice and lentil casserole.

SOME SNACK SELECTIONS
Any fresh fruit. Matzo with jelly/jam. Toast and jelly/jam. Baked potato, vegetable sticks, cucumber/zucchini slices, pickles, muffins, bagels. Popcorn, baked apple, non-fat milk cocoa, fruit juices, vegetable juices. Lentil soup with brown bread. Beer, wine, walnuts.

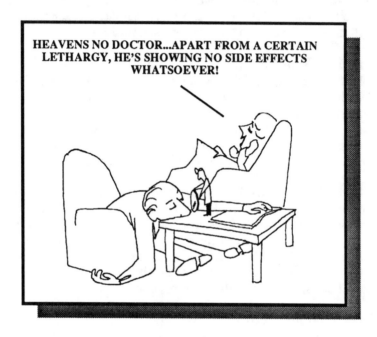

4 | BLOOD PRESSURE ACTION STEPS

DOES HIGH BLOOD PRESSURE ALWAYS MEAN PILLS?

YOU MIGHT CONSIDER THESE ALTERNATIVES...

1) LESS SALT

Philadelphia researchers modified the salt intakes of a population of blood pressure patients by having them avoid processed and fast foods and by adding no salt in the kitchen or at the table. No salt at the table cuts out about 1 teaspoon a day. No salt in the cooking cuts out another teaspoon. These moves cut sodium intakes by 2/3 and blood pressures by 10% to 20%.

An Australian study demonstrated that adding 2 vegetables a day decreased the blood pressure of untreated patients with moderate hypertension without any change in their weights or any attention to salt.

WHERE'S THE SALT?

Ketchup / pickles / relish / mustard / dressings / canned soups / sauces / gravies / packaged soups / fast foods / restaurant foods / microwaved dinners / smoked-cured meats / chips / packaged cereals & snacks / cakes / pies / cookies / rolls / pizza / cheese / instant puddings / etc.

Any food that reaches you straight from the ground is low in sodium, high in potassium and very good for you. Many are called vegetables.

2) WEIGHT CONTROL

Chicago researchers reported in 1990 that a maintained weight loss of only 10 pounds, or cutting daily salt intakes by 1/3, or cutting alcohol intakes in half restored 40% of mild to moderate hypertensive patients to normal. Among the remaining 60%, such intervention lowered the pressures of most even if complete normalcy was not attained.

WHERE'S WEIGHT CONTROL?

In a foodstyle that's low in fat and high in fiber and a lifestyle of fitness that gets your resting heart rate down to fewer than 60 beats per minute. In addition to weighing yourself, learn to check your pulse rate (need a watch) and your pressure (need a cuff).

3) FITNESS

In the nation's executive suites, blood pressures go up with megabuck risks and are accompanied by other stress signs: anxiety and anger. Different executives develop different ways to manage their challenges. Some let off steam by snapping at subordinates but alternative mechanisms are even more effective. Like working it off. Studies of executive urine outputs of adrenalin indicate that fit executives are less stressed than their sedentary colleagues. Risk-taking and risk-making are action situations that produce action moods, so the blood pressure goes up to provide a better circulation to the muscles.

Another study of hypertension in Australia revealed a remarkable effect of alcohol. Among hypertensive men consuming more than 2 servings of alcohol a day, cutting their intakes in half without any other intervention, also cut their elevated blood pressure levels in half.

WHERE'S FITNESS?

It begins with 5 miles a week on foot covering a mile in 15 minutes, continues in a measurably beneficial way to 10 miles to 15 to 20 to 25. Beyond 25 miles week on foot no greater heart, pressure,or health benefits can be measured.

HYPERTENSION CONTROL CHECKLIST

TOWARD POORER HEALTH

☐ DAILY ALCOHOL

☐ DAILY FAST FOOD FARE

☐ DAILY RESTAURANT FARE

☐ DAILY PACKAGED SNAX & PUDDINGS , DESSERTS

TOWARD BETTER HEALTH

☐ OCCASIONAL ALCOHOL

☐ A CLEANER CUISINE

☐ DISCOVERY OF HERBS AND SPICES

☐ SEVERAL VEGETABLES DAILY

☐ BIOSTRESS MANAGEMENT BASICS

☐ DAILY BRISK WALKS

COACH'S CORNER

SALTING UP THE PRESSURE

People with high blood pressure often seem to have no problems and no complaints for years. Eventually, however, high blood pressure causes excess cholesterol to accumulate in heart arteries for a heart attack, or the pumping heart to fail because it has been working too
hard against increased pressure for too long, or the high pressure to cause ballooning of an artery in the brain where it may burst with bleeding into the brain to produce a stroke.

World-wide, the highest incidence of high blood pressure and strokes is to be found in northern Japan where the salt intake is extreme (twice as high as ours). By way of contrast, 20 countries around the world with very low salt intakes (half as high as ours) have practically no high blood pressure and no bursting strokes.

Where salt is scarce high blood pressure is scarce, and where salt is in wide-spread use, high blood pressure is common. Salt does not cause high blood pressure in everybody, but aggravates any inherited, natural tendency.

193

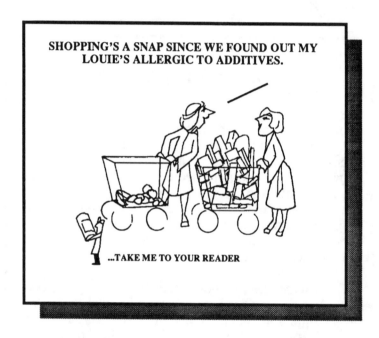

5 FOOD SENSITIVITY ACTION STEPS

NEED A FIELD GUIDE
TO FOOD SENSITIVITIES?

CONSIDER THIS
JUMP START

Probably a third of us suffer from unrecognized food sensitivities: vague daylong aches and pains, food cravings, itchings and swellings, sinus congestion, fatigue and depression, headache or digestive complaints. The list is growing. And the foods responsible are not always frivolous foods like chocolate and sugar, but serious foods like milk, wheat, corn, eggs, even chicken or fish.

These are still generally unrecognized clinical discoveries for several reasons. First, there's no reliable laboratory test; and skin tests don't work for foods for most people. Perhaps food gets changed by the digestive process into problem items. Skin tests show inhalants well (pollens etc.), but not ingestants. Second, the symptoms produced by food often take one to three days to appear, so late that no association with the food is made. And third, symptoms often get worse during the first few days that the offending food is withheld.

So you must become attuned to your own body. Watch your lungs for example. Are they producing extra mucus? Do they wheeze when you twist your chest by swinging your arms with your mouth open? Minor degrees of food sensitivity can cause airway irritation without asthma. Minor sensitivities can cause vague abdominal discomforts, aches without severe cramps. Poke your fingertips into your belly. You should be as comfortable in the belly as you are from the same poke into the muscle of your thigh. Tenderness means trouble.

Study your stools. Pellets of stool, say the size of beans or golf balls, such stools indicate a gut going into painless or achy spasm. Something in your diet is not agreeing with you. Much constipation is a result of unrecognized food sensitivity.

It's very easy, beware, with all this encouraged and necessary introspection to become neurotic, so don't underestimate the power of your imagination to cause or to exaggerate your symptoms. On the other hand, don't ignore the power of your mind to deny such symptoms.

STEP 1

THE EXCLUSION PHASE
A TIME OF HEALING

To determine just what foods are causing you problems, confine your eating to the following selection for two weeks. It's not a diet for weight control so eat any amount you wish. Weight loss will often occur from the several pounds of water in the fluid of inflammation in your tissues.

Do not eat any food or drink any items that are not identified on the list of options below. Eat no mixture of foods, and no canned or processed foods unless you know all the ingredients and they are on the list below. Take no alcohol and no aspirin. For aches and pains use Tylenol.

Feeling poorly over the first few days is a good sign. It means your system is clearing itself of toxic products. By the second week you should feel as though a storm has passed and you're in the clear.

USUAL EXCLUSION DIET SELECTIONS

BEVERAGES: water, tea, grape juice and pineapple juice- no sugar added.

CEREALS: oatmeal or rice without milk and served with any juice above.

BREADS: Rye Crisp plain, barley plain, rye or potato flour bread.

FATS: olive oil only for cooking or salads.

FRUITS: grapes, apricots, plums, cherries, pineapples, apples.

MEATS: lamb or well-done beef - not pink but gray.

VEGETABLES: carrots, beets, olives, celery, beet greens, yams, lettuce, white potatoes, broccoli - flavor with salt or olive oil only, no herbs or pepper or spices.

SEASONINGS: salt, ginger, vanilla extract, cinnamon.

SWEETENERS: Nutrasweet or honey.

THE EXCLUSION DIET DAILY MENU

FOR BREAKFASTS TRY:
Bowl of puffed rice cereal with pineapple. Allowed juice/fruit/tea. Oatmeal cooked in water topped with honey or no-sugar-added applesauce or Nutrasweet. Bowl of brown rice topped with honey or applesauce. Allowed fruit/fruit juice/tea.

FOR LUNCHES TRY:
Sandwich consisting of pure rye bread, lettuce, and roast beef or lamb loaf, plus celery, and carrot sticks. Salad consisting of all or any of the following: lettuce, beets, shredded carrots, olives, broccoli, celery and shredded beef. Olive oil salad dressing. Rye Crisps.

FOR DINNERS TRY:
Lamb stew (see recipe). Barley biscuits (see recipe). Applesauce and allowed fruit/fruit juice/tea/water. Beef with steamed rice, carrots and broccoli stir fry. Tossed salad - lettuce, beets, olives, celery, salad dressing. Tapioca pudding (see recipe). Lamb loaf (see recipe). Mashed potatoes, steamed carrots.

FOR SNACKS TRY:
Rice cakes with honey or applesauce. Barley biscuits (see recipe). Tapioca pudding (see recipe). Rye Crisps, Rye toast, carrot and celery sticks. Allowed fruit/fruit juice.

STEP 2
THE CHALLENGE PHASE
A TIME OF DETECTION

While on the Exclusion diet, challenge yourself with foods from the list below. These are the most common causes of food sensitivity, but the list is not complete.

To eliminate guesswork, begin to assemble a list of foods for you that are OK FOODS, NOT OK FOODS and MAYBE FOODS.   During this transition state of food challenge you must remain on the Exclusion Diet while eating servings of the particular challenge food. Be on the lookout for your own particular pattern of symptoms. Common symptoms include: **Any morning you wake up with a headache, a stuffed nose or feeling like you've got the flu without a fever, you probably ate something the day before to which you're sensitive.**

If you develop symptoms after a single challenge exposure, stop the challenge right there.   And always wait until symptoms have cleared before you challenge yourself with a new item.   Foods that don't provoke symptoms after several challenges over two days (followed by a 3 day watching period for delayed reactions) are probably safe and can be added to the OK FOODS list and incorporated into your basic Exclusion Diet. Crowding challenges too closely together can lead to confusion.

A CHALLENGE RECORD

Write in how you felt after each challenge (up to 48 hours), your symptoms, when they happened and how long they lasted.

COW'S MILK FOODS
Any milk (two glasses a day), cheese, yogurt, cream or butter

---

WHEAT FOODS
Any wheat cereal (shredded wheat, puffed wheat), breads, rolls, buns

---

EGG FOODS
Any cooked egg, (two a day any way, yolk and white), chicken too

---

CORN FOODS
Corn flakes, chips, pop corn, corn flour, corn syrup, corn oil

---

CITRUS FOODS
Oranges, grapefruit, lemon, lime, citrus-flavored soda pop

SUGAR FOODS
Cane sugar, candy, cakes, pies, beet sugar, syrup, regular pop

---

CHOCOLATE FOODS
Chocolate candy, chocolate milk, cocoa, cola drinks, chocolate syrup

---

YEAST / MOLDS
Wine, beer, cider, yeast baked goods, cheese, mushrooms, supplements

---

FOODS THAT DO NOT OFTEN
CAUSE SENSITIVITY REACTIONS

The following foods might help you quickly develop a list of OK FOODS.

apples	apricots	asparagus
avocado	beets	barley
brussel sprouts	carrots	cauliflower
celery	chicken	coffee
cranberries	dates	dried beans
eggplant	frog legs	garlic
gingerale	grapes	lamb
honey	lobster	lettuce
olive oil	oats	peas
pea pods	pineapple	pepper
potato	rabbit	radishes
raisins	rice	rye flour
safflower oil	salmon	soy products
spices	spinach	sprouts
squash	sunflower seeds	sweet potatoes
tea	tapioca	turkey
vanilla extract	yams	zucchini

By keeping records (eventually your memory will serve), offending foods can be uncovered and identified. Although sensitivities tend to recede with time, you are dealing with a moving target and changing conditions. You must begin to read your dials. **Beware of foods that you feel strongly about.**

FOOD SENSITIVITY CHECKLIST

TOWARD POORER HEALTH

☐ MORNING HEADACHES, SINUS-NASAL STUFFINESS

☐ MORNING TENDERNESS: EYES, BELLY, MUSCLES, JOINTS

☐ MORNING SWELLINGS: FACE, HANDS, FINGERS, WEIGHT UP

TOWARD BETTER HEALTH

☐ DAIRY CHECK: ESPECIALLY CHEESE

☐ GRAIN CHECK: ESPECIALLY WHEAT OR CORN PRODUCTS

☐ MOLD CHECK: ESPECIALLY WINE OR BEER

☐ RESTAURANT CHECK: ESPECIALLY SOUPS AND SAUCES

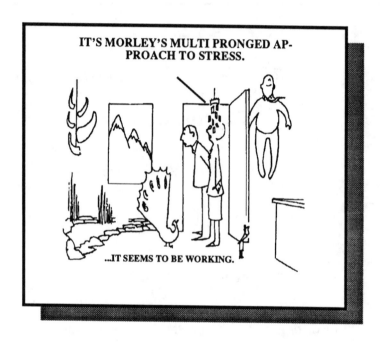

6 | BIOSTRESS ACTION STEPS

WANT A FIELD GUIDE
TO BIOSTRESS?

...CONSIDER
THIS JUMP START

Stress is a pain, a mood pain and not a physical pain, but still a pain; and because avoiding pain is a law of life, stress produces feelings we try to avoid or be rid of. That was its survival effect, it forced us to take action, to get comfortable, to stay alive. But a pain-free life is impossible because pain is protective.

Stress starts in the brain, a 3-pound lump of nerves, numbering about 15 billion or more, each with about 10,000 connections. It's an enormously complex coordinating system, one of several in the body, with its own evolutionary history. There's an old, indeed ancient, part of the brain, the bottom half that's responsible for most of the expressions of stress. There's also a more recent, intelligent new part.

The old part, Old Brain, is at the bottom. The new part, New Brain, is at the top. The old part is older than the new part by millions of years, but New Brain makes us human and intellectual. Old Brain is where we feel things, where we react to threats. Its the Department of Defense and its reactions to perceived threats constitute the phenomenon of stress. So stress is an unpleasant feeling, produced by changes in our world that are perceived to be threats. Our reactions to perceived threats constitute the phenomenon of stress.

The perception of threat usually starts in New Brain, from which signals pass down to Old Brain to produce a response that's rooted in a biology millions of years old. Today's threats, however, are seldom threats to life as they once were. They're usually threats to expectations or plans, to income or personal relations. Yet the response they trigger is keyed to physical threats, to life and death survival. That's what stress is and what it's all about ... running and fighting, fear and anger; flight or fight, anxiety or aggravation.

By recognizing this interplay of New and Old Brain we can apply our intelligence (New) to the task of managing fear and rage (Old). We can intellectualize mood mangement for better outcomes and the first step in this process is

206

understanding demands and performance in tissue terms.

Nearly 100 years ago, researchers working with the heart demonstrated a basic principle of biological behavior. Increasing the workload leads to an increase in performance, but only up to a point. Expressed as a curve representing the plot of rising demands against responsive performance, the curve at first slopes sharply upwards then gradually flattens and sharply declines.

LOAD-PERFORMANCE OR DEMAND-RESPONSE CURVE

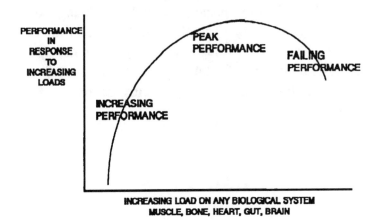

Although the curve was derived from observations on the isolated heart, as a phenomenon it applies to all biological behavior, mental and physical. A simple example of both at the same time would be to imagine a telephone answering assignment. There are several incoming lines and your job is to represent the organization courteously, answer inquiries satisfactorily, manage complaints tactfully and forward incoming orders expeditiously. As the volume ebbs and flows your performance matches demands. Increased incoming calls (demands) are met by increased forwarding, answering, reassuring and accommodating (response) so that a plot of events would reveal a rising demand-performance curve.

So far so good. You know your job, the calls come in at a rate of one every 5-10 minutes, and take a few minutes to manage. You are all sweetness and light cascading from a gracious height upon one and all. But the pace of the calls increases. They now average one every 3 minutes and at times several lines are flashing. In addition, one of your new product lines has quality problems, so many of the calls are complaints.

DEMAND-RESPONSE CURVE
WITH MOODS INCLUDED

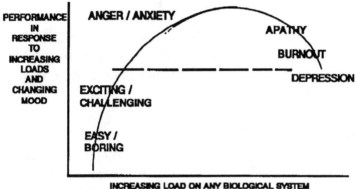

The interrupted line represents the threshold below which stress is not felt, so stress management must take into account changing the threshold. It can vary from moment to moment or day to day, depending on you and your body.

At some point in your performance, your capacity is not impaired but an unpleasant mood of tension or irritation creeps in. You are now stressed. Later your response begins to flatten out, not quite as efficient or easy, and your mood passes from challenge to aggravation to indifference as you get overwhelmed and retreat in psychological self defense. From a mood of confidence, you become anxious, uncertain and less accommodating. Performance may be maintained early on, but at a cost, and your new mood we call stress.

Two basic performance-protecting strategies that emerge from this understanding of biological systems involve managing demands and managing performance.

The first strategy must address inputs: managing the day's workload, the system's demands. And the second strategy must address your reactions: Managing the body, its brain and tissues, the system response.

When demands can be met readily and performed easily, our mood is one of quiet confidence. As demands call for greater skill (and less certainty of outcome) moods of excitement and challenge begin to be felt. This is where most of us function best and would like to spend our working days. The horizontal line represents an emotional threshold below which we feel alive, lively and productive; and above which (even while more productive) our mood has shifted to one of tension and aggravation. Eventually performance flattens and then falls as moods of fatigue, indifference and depression set in.

Ideally, one is most productive when at that point on the curve just below its first intercept with the threshold for anger or anxiety, where challenge is the mood and performance is good. From this perspective, 3 strategies suggest themselves to achieve that end; strategies that reduce your position along the demand ordinate or raise the threshold of tolerance. First, whenever and wherever possible reduce inputs so they don't overwhelm your response. Second, raise your tolerance threshold physically through wellness activities. And third, raise your threshold mentally, through relaxation techniques.

GETTING SOMETHING OFF YOUR CHEST
RARELY GETS IT OFF YOUR BACK

SO STOP IT

There's a convenient memory device based on the demand-performance curve and your own sensitivity to that threshold where your ability to deal comfortably with demands has been passed.

The mnemonic device is called "Stop It," two words of an affirmation that should come naturally to mind as you feel yourself growing tense or irritated. **STOP IT** provides a short hand, mental review mechanism for rationally assessing ways to reduce demands or raise your threshold of tolerance for them as they arise in your day or life.

STOP-IT

S   Squeeze something. Do something physical. Now. Squeeze your fists or your knees together. Anything. Smile. Stretch.

T   Talk, tranquilize. Do something mental now... Visualize. Imagine. Pray. Affirm. Sing. Whistle. Recite.

O   Open it up. Do something physical later. Soak. Work-out. Write. Call someone. Run. Dance. Shout. Sing. Scream. Swear.

P   Play around. Do something mental later. Music. Week-end retreat. Visit friends, relatives. Hobbies. Books. Tapes. Films.

I   Impose controls. Close some doors. Prioritize. Dismiss. Reject. Move along. Grow. Eliminate toxic habits, attitudes. Review obligations. Learn to say no!

T   Take another tack. Open some doors... new people, places, activities, goals, job skills. Share. Delegate. Communicate.

213

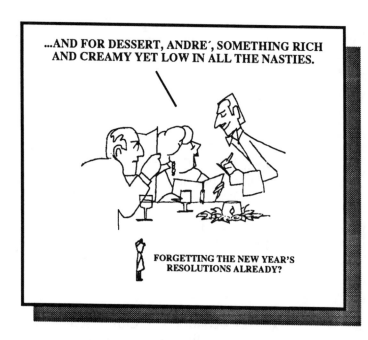

7   OVERWEIGHT ACTION STEPS

THE NATIONAL WEIGHT PROBLEM:

SOME REFLECTIONS AND A JUMP START

Like any basic human behavior, feeding behavior can get distorted too. We all binge now and then, indulging in a food gorge, an episode of excess: At Thanksgiving perhaps; in a depressed mood; or to celebrate. Binge eating can be triggered by outside influences such as the sight or scent of food, or from inside influences such as hunger, fatigue, anxiety anger; or combinations. Or something else. Such as? An itch.

For many binge eaters there's nothing wrong with their food intake systems. It's the signal to stop, the sense of satiety or fullness that fails them. The sense of contentment or satiety that normally comes with food eludes them because food satisfaction is not the satisfaction they need. Like an itch that won't go away and can't be reached for satisfactory relief, they're scratching around the spot until they bleed. Many such individuals have developed a sensitivity or "allergy" to the very foods they crave.

For other individuals food is a comfort, and those who turn to food are not weight-prone, experience no penalty for their comfort eating. The extra calories will be incinerated spontaneously as they usually are when lean people over-eat, so their compensation or comfort eating tends to go unnoticed. But individuals turning to food for comfort who are weight-prone (as half the population is) have a weight gain, a penalty to show or perhaps to avoid. And you avoid at all costs if you are a young woman in our culture.

Studies from the University of Cincinnati suggest that binge eating and vomiting are not rare on today's college campuses. Perhaps 20% of female undergraduates practice it on occasion. It's a habit they resort to, to minimize weight gain after over-eating, but carries a risk of mineral depletion, of aspiration , vomit into the lungs, or of tearing of the tube that connects mouth and stomach.

More fiber in the diet would help return appetite to its roots and their satisfaction. Fiber provokes chewing (a demonstrated source of appetite satisfaction), expands the stomach (another source), and delays absorption (another

216

source). Fiber also traps calories and prevents their absorption. A calorie may be a calorie, but food is the source of the these calories and physiology is the means of their use and storage. So sometimes a calorie is not a calorie when you look at the physiology. Take for example, a study done on peanuts. Eating peanuts as peanut butter leads to 97% of the peanut calories being absorbed, but by eating the nuts of peanut butter as peanuts only 85% of the calories are absorbed. That's due to the vagaries of fiber and chewing and digestion.

> *"FOODS ARE HANDLED AND THEIR CALORIES DISTRIBUTED DIFFERENTLY AT DIFFERENT TIMES OF THE DAY."*

Beyond these vagaries of absorption and assimilation, calories are also utilized differently at different times in the day, in the cycle of our daily clocks. Calories are swept up and burned at times of tissue maintenance and repair; and when muscle energy expenditure is at its peak. That's during the waking hours. At other times, calories are more likely to be stored as fat. So the message for weight-prone individuals from those studies is to spread your calories over the day and not have them lumped toward the end.

Studies from Texas have shown what a bad deal end of day calories are. Six healthy adults, three male and three female, consumed a single 2,000-calorie meal in the morning each day for 1 week. Then they ate the same meal in the evening each day for a week. All other activities over the weeks of the study were sedentary and similar, but the results were different. All subjects lost weight when they took their calories at the beginning of the day, while four of the six gained weight when they took their calories at the end of the day. Their clocks were ticking. Thanks to body clocks and their effect on metabolism, a meal eaten at breakfast is less likely to get converted to fat than the same meal eaten late in the day.

There are dozens of clocks in all of us. They tick away and time events: Simple events such as waking and sleeping or complex events such as feeding and hunger. They involve the very rhythm of existence and are beginning to provide grist for the mills of obesity research. In the clinic it's been known for decades that sugar and protein are handled differently in the body from morning to afternoon in the same person. A normal glucose tolerance test in the morning often becomes abnormal in the afternoon. Foods are handled and their calories distributed differently at different times of the day.

The message of the Texas study is that a large food intake toward the end of the day, even one within your calorie budget, is disastrous to weight control. It sets you up for storage. Yet you can't face the prospect of a full breakfast; you say, so perhaps snacking is the way: nibbling no more than 50 or 100 calories of food every 2-3 hours through the day, fueling the furnace that keeps you warm and the engine that moves you around, rather than filling your fuel tanks with fat.

"...EATING SMALLER AMOUNTS AT MORE FREQUENT INTERVALS, GIVING UP GORGING FOR GRAZING."

So there are several lessons from science in all these observations that can help with weight control. The lessons involve avoiding artificial sweeteners, eating more high fiber foods, eating more of our food earlier in the day, and eating smaller amounts at more frequent intervals, giving up gorging for grazing.

THE FASTING JUMP START

A total fast involves taking no calories, no food and drinking only non-caloric fluids (no calories such as fruit juice). It should be medically supervised. For most individuals seeking the benefits of fasting however, a partial or modified fast is less demanding, and begins to get the job done. It is undertaken with a view to controlling ketone production, that is to say, controlling the production of smoke from burning fat by taking carbohydrate over the day in the form of fruit juice. In excess amounts ketones in the blood can make you nauseous.

Misgivings over fasting are less medical than psychological. Going without food for long periods is, in fact, a natural state. We have become so conditioned by abundance as to be afraid to go without food, to go hungry. Among individuals who practice fasting, most have recorded comments that are supportive and enthusiastic, such as: "It really clears the head by the second week." "It's my money-saving spa alternative." "I understand its religious associations ... there's a definite mental lift that's almost transcendental." Such comments are common in the literature on fasting and provide some insight into reasons that its practitioners see the practice as the opportunity for a restoration of feelings and chemistry and body weight to better levels at intervals throughout their lives.

220

During a modified fast, total fluid intake over the day should exceed several quarts. It's purpose is to wash the metabolites of tissue burning out of your blood so they don't accumulate and cause mischief. Over the day, at 3 hour intervals, a tumbler of fruit or vegetable juice helps keep body chemistry on the rails. From 18 to 36 ounces of juice over the day usually do the job.

Fasting takes at least 2 weeks for any significant body benefit, and ideally 3 or 4 weeks. Fasting breaks many compulsive behaviors regarding food such as cravings and binge eating. It decongests fat cells which is the reason it has such a prompt and beneficial effect on high blood sugars. It sharpens the senses and lifts the mood and has a calming effect on behavior. Fasting is sometimes the first nutrient tool for self discipline. With the open time that is created, opportunities arise to read and reflect, go for walks, put your mental house in order, write letters, keep a journal, contact old friends, listen to music, meditate and even enjoy some spiritual reflection. It's also quite compatible with a productive work load. Away from work, bicycle rides around the neighborhood or a soak or a swim or working around the yard and the garden, painting, sculpting, beading or hobbying. Avoid vigorous effort however, because the biggest problem is that you become fatigued and easily irritated.

Toward the end of the fast be prepared to take it easy. And because elevated blood pressures come down,

221

lightheadedness especially after getting up from a recumbent position is a common complaint. It's not a bad sign but simply a signal to get up slowly after you have been lying down. A coated tongue should be brushed regularly when you brush your teeth because it's not being scrapped clean with food as is the normal circumstance.

Finally, come back from your fast gently with small food portions...bowls of soups or salads without dressing. During this return to food time, rediscover vegetables, whether steamed, microwaved or raw. You'll be surprised to discover what a sharp flavor they provide, far sharper than you remember.

Warning: In the 1970s, dozens of deaths were reported among people placing themselves on an unsupervised, protein-drink modified fast. If you think that a juice modified fast for 2 - 4 weeks might help you, first get a second opinion. Ask your physician if there is any reason it could pose problems for you, and if not would your physician would be willing to supervise you ? then follow the advice you get.

DIETS GET IT DOWN
FITNESS KEEPS IT THERE

WINNING THE WELLNESS GAME

A WEIGHT CONTROL CHECKLIST

TOWARD POORER HEALTH

☐ HIGH FAT FOODS: MEATS, DAIRIES, OILS AND SPREADS

☐ LOW FIBER FOODS: JUICES, ENRICHED FLOURS , PKGED. SNAX

☐ SEDENTARY WAYS: DES KS , DRIVING, TELEVIEWING

TOWARD BETTER HEALTH

☐ LEAN MEAT, SPRINKLE CHEESE, FAT SUSTITUTES

☐ DISCOVER DAILY VEGETABLES

☐ POPCORN SNAX, FRESH FRUIT SNAX

☐ DAILY BRISK WALKS

☐ SINGLE ITEM ALL-YOU- WANT FOOD ENCOUNTERS

☐ CANNED FRUIT/VEGETABLE WORKBREAKS

☐ 6 - 8 DAILY FOOD ENCOUNTERS OF ABOUT 150 CALS EACH

223

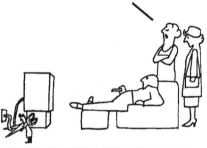

FITNESS ACTION STEPS

BUT I'M NOT COORDINATED

...THEN WALKING IS YOUR GAME

Feet strike the ground about a thousand times apiece each mile of a walk or run, so they take a pounding over any distance. It makes sense to wear comfortable sox and properly designed, good-fitting shoes. Even the fanciest of today's fancy shoes cost less than a dime a mile, which is hardly an expensive trip.

A good walking or jogging shoe is cushioned to help absorb road shock which can be tough on ankles, knees and hips as well as feet. Good training shoes absorb up to a third of the road shock, thanks to built-in layers of cushion.

In addition to the cushion, good shoes have a supporting cup built-in around the heel. Often made of plastic, it's called a counter, and provides lateral stability, reducing heel wobble at the moment of contact with the road. Excess heel wobble can lead to knee and ankle problems over the miles.

Body weight is normally distributed along the outside edge of the sole of the foot during a walk or run. The natural arch of the normal foot assures this distribution of weight and to promote it, good shoes have arch cushions built under the insole. Look for them inside the shoe.

Look for a soft roll of binding along the mouth of the shoe and a tab rise over the heel. They help reduce irritation of the skin around the ankle and protect the Achilles tendon. Whether shoe uppers are of nylon or thin leather is of little performance consequence. The colors and designs are now so darling as to threaten traditional locker room ambiance.

Walking and running are basically simple, natural, even sweaty activities; childish exuberances that call for a step or two of adult caution in the selection of foot wear. But there's a world of helpful technology at your feet. A dozen top line shoes are competing aggressively for your trade with designer colors and fiercely tricky minor marketing advantages. If the shoe that catches your fancy has the supportive features mentioned, try it on. If it fits and feels good, do it. And have a look at some of the smart outfits available too. Make a statement about your commitment.

FOR JOINTS

The possibility that regular fitness activities might wear out the hips or knees continues to nag doctors recommending exercise to their patients. A California study in 1985 on 55 runners is reassuring. It was an intensive evaluation of runners who had run at least 10,000 miles over a 5 year period. They were compared to matched non-running controls and found to have healthier, denser bones. There was no sign of cartilage loss or wear-and-tear arthritis.

A similar 5-year study in Florida involved a smaller group of older runners with the same results. At an average age of 53, they ran 30 miles a week and were found to have a lower incidence of wear-and-tear arthritis. They also enjoyed better overall health and had fewer disabilities than a comparable group of same-age, non-runner controls.

AND FOR BONES

The fragile bones of osteoporosis are of general concern to many women today, and after examining 300 women between the ages of 18 and 75, orthopedic surgeons in North Carolina determined that active women over the age of 50 had tougher, healthier bones than did women who didn't exercise regularly.

227

PRELIMINARY CONSIDERATIONS

For fitness to become a habit and its benefits to become part of the way you feel and live, the effort it requires must be made as simple, convenient and pleasant as possible. And that means making time, making plans and avoiding pain. You should be weather proofed for the seasons with appropriate colorful, protective gear.

Don't ignore today's entertainment possibilities if you prefer not to be with your thoughts. There are headset radios and tape players, for company there are spas, fitness clubs, walking clubs, malls and neighbors or friends, even a dog. For record-keeping, there are pedometers, timers, workbooks, calendars and treadmills.

Any time is a good time to go for a walk so fit it into the other demands of your day. To make time, go to bed half an hour earlier, start your day half an hour earlier and use that half hour for fitness. Evening walking is better than none at all but it juices you up before bed time which is going against the grain. Although it's most satisfying to shower after a brisk walk, few workplaces permit the time or opportunity midday. Toweling in the rest room works because fresh sweat doesn't smell. The basic daily unit of fitness is a mile in 15 minutes without discomfort, and with enough breath left over to whistle, sing, or chat.

A PERFORMANCE GUIDE FOR BEGINNERS

TAKE 1-6 WEEKS
TO GO FROM 10 MINUTES A DAY TO 30

THEN TAKE ANOTHER 1-6 WEEKS
TO GO FROM 1 MILE IN 20 MINUTES TO 2
MILES IN 30 MINUTES

THEN TAKE ANOTHER 1-6 WEEKS
TO GO FROM 3 MILES IN AN HOUR
TO 4 MILES IN AN HOUR
FIVE TIMES A WEEK.

ACHES AND PAINS

Overuse injuries are the most common complication of recovering fitness. They must be expected because they are the rule and not the exception. They are a signal to rest, cut back, heal and pick it up again. For persistent problems see your doctor or a fitness expert.

THE MOST COMMON FITNESS PROBLEMS

MUSCLE SORENESS: Usually a result of tiny muscle fiber tears. Rest and cold first day. Rest and heat subsequent days.

MUSCLE CRAMPS: An overused muscle contracts and stays knotted. Rest, massage and gentle stretching.

MUSCLE STRAIN: Usually a result of larger muscle fiber tears. Rest and cold first day. Rest and heat subsequent days.

SIDE STITCH: Thought to be due to spasm of a segment of the diaphragm. Slow down. Stop. Rest.

TENDON/LIGAMENT SPRAIN: Torn fibrous tissue around joint at end of muscle. Rest and cold first day. Rest and heat subsequent day. Slower to heal than muscle.

SHIN SPLINTS: Catchall term for tenderness in the front of the leg. Usually muscle tears, sometimes stress fracture. Rest and cold first day. Rest and heat subsequent days. Get help if not resolving in few days.

CALF PAIN: Usually overuse but in older individual may signal circulation problem. Cut back, rest, heal. Get advice.

HEEL PAIN: Usually a bruised point and not a "spur". The "spur" is not a spur at all. It is a fleck of painless calcium in an old blood clot from long ago. The pain and tenderness are from continuing tendon and ligament tears around the area. Find the tender spot, and mark the point with felt-tipped pen, then, without sox, walk in shoes with an inserted foam insole, cut out the stained patch and re-insert insole. Wear for 1-2 weeks of healing.

ARCH PAIN: Usually torn planter ligaments on sole of foot. Rest, cold first day. Rest, heat subsequent days. Consider arch support over the counter or professional prosthetic made to fit.

231

ACHILLES TENDONITIS: Tenderness along the major heel tendon. An overuse problem. Rest and cold first day. Rest and heat subsequent days.

KNEE INJURY: Usually torn supporting outside ligaments or inside(cruciate) ligaments. Rest and cold first day. Get professional help if not responding. A very vulnerable joint.

HIP INJURY: As for the knee. Rest and hot baths. Get professional help early rather than late.

LOWER BACK ACHES: Usually a racquet sport or old contact injury. Rest and cold first day. Rest and heat thereafter. Get professional help. Consider a regular program of back strengthening exercises. The American back is in general a vulnerable back from a lifetime of physical inactivity that leads to back muscle wasting. The two muscles that run down your back on either side of your spine should be as well developed as your forearm. Have a look in the bathroom mirror.

A FITNESS CHECKLIST

TOWARD POORER HEALTH

- [ ] CAR COMMUTING
- [ ] DESK INCOME
- [ ] DAILY TELEVIEWING
- [ ] RECREATIONAL GADGETS

TOWARD BETTER HEALTH

- [ ] DAILY BRISK WALKS AT LEAST 20 MINUTES
- [ ] DAILY BRISK WALKS HEART RATE UP TO 100 PER MINUTE
- [ ] DAILY PRECAUTION WITH THE TALK TEST
- [ ] WEEKLY HOT SPOTS CHECK
- [ ] WEEKLY EQUIPMENT CHECK
- [ ] WEEKLY MOOD/INTEREST SUPPORT
- [ ] WEEKLY LOG/RECORD PERFORMANCE CHECK

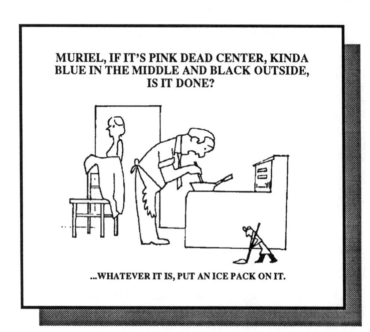

CLEAN CUISINE ACTION STEPS

BUT COOKING'S NOT FOR ME!

...THEN THIS JUMP START IS

The road to wellness has many potholes. On one occasion I joined a panel of wellness experts on Detroit television for a review of health and fitness. I looked forward to a discussion of the issues, differences of opinion probably, and the arrival at some agreeable consensus.

At the studio, however I met an attractive young woman and two men in sober business suits. Could these be my fellow panelists, I wondered? No, I was told, only the woman. All three were representatives of a national fast food chain but the woman was a **Registered Dietitian**, and only she would appear on the show. The men I realized, were riding shotgun, reinforcing off-camera any tendency to stray from party lines. During the show I wore what I thought was a warm and attentive smile, although I did feel it freeze into place. The woman went on and on about the importance of a balanced diet.   Nothing was bad in moderation. Cheeseburgers and fries can be redeemed with a little high fiber lettuce and tomato on the side.

I was in a quandary. To counter with rude facts some of her "balanced" diet pieties, would leave me looking the sexist pig out in viewer land. So I murmured something mellow and evasive on cue, eventually leaving the studio somewhat depressed.   It was another in a string of aggravating experiences with official health agencies, food processors and even those among my colleagues who have been slow to accept the accumulating data.

We're living through a period that will probably be looked back upon as the Century of Nutrition. During its first 50 years we learned the science of safe infant feeding and minimal adult nutrient needs. We learned about vitamins, and minerals and calories and protein. During the second half of this century (since World War II) we have discovered the health hazards of excess. In 1988, the U.S. Surgeon General published a report on nutrition. It was the first time for such a publication in the hundred year history of the office. In the sense of full health after 40, wellness these days is rarely an accident. And the first steps begin in the kitchen.

First, face the stove. It's where you're going to apply a little heat to food, and that's about it. You'll also need some pots, some covered dishes, a freezer and a fridge.

236

SHOPPING THE WALLS

Try to shop on a full stomach, and preferably, alone. Once in the store, stick to your list. It's estimated that 50% of purchased food is bought on impulse and food bought impulsively is the kind you don't need. Retailers attempt to increase impulse buying by displaying the most expensive and always the most processed foods at eye level. These foods almost always contain excess amounts of fat, salt and sugar. Rather than browse up and down the aisles of the store, shop the outer edge. Here you'll find fruits, vegetables, dairy products, breads, chicken, and fish.

Choose products low in fat. In the dairy department this means selecting skim milk or skim cottage cheese. Try to steer clear of cheese. If you must, use pungent cheeses such as Feta, Romano, Parmesan or Bleu in your recipes. Salad dressings which are almost all fat, can be replaced with No-Oil dressing.

In the bread and pasta department, think whole wheat. Choose breads with the first ingredient listed as whole wheat flour. Use whole wheat pasta and flour, as well as brown rice and other whole grains, to further increase your intake of fiber. Fruits and vegetables are good sources of fiber.

BATCH COOKING BASICS

Make it a point while putting groceries away to scrub and repackage as many items as feasible to make them easier to deal with later. For example, fill the sink with soapy water and allow apples and other edible-skin fruit to soak while you are busy elsewhere. A quick rub, rinse, and a few minutes in the dish strainer means that they are ready to be stored in a large bowl on the counter or packaged into one handy container, or into several small "single encounter" sized ones. A bag of carrots can be scrubbed and repackaged as a unit, or cut up and packaged in baggies for lunches and snack encounters. Also, take a minute to package the vegetables you'll need for each of the week's recipes or meals in the same bag. A carrot, stalk of broccoli, and sweet pepper, scrubbed and ready to go, can be stored together for a stir-fry. Break packages of poultry into recipe-sized units before refrigerating or freezing.

Set aside a time each week to cook up large batches of base foods, such as brown rice, beans, sauces, and dressings. Package them in sizes that fit your recipes, and store. Beans, rice and many sauces freeze beautifully, while salad dressings are best refrigerated. Frozen rice can be quickly defrosted in a vegetable steamer and used with stir-fried vegetables or under sauces. Or, drop the frozen rice into a pot of soup. Beans take longer to thaw, so take them out in the morning to thaw or defrost in the microwave oven.

SEASONING WITHOUT SALT

You have a variety of seasonings to choose from other than salt. Flavored vinegars, lemon juice, wine, liquors, Parmesan cheese, fresh or dried herbs, and spices are a few examples. Start out with fresh and dried herbs and spices by using them sparingly.

Dried herbs are stronger, so use about 1/4 teaspoon of dried herbs for each teaspoon of fresh. After you've become familiar with their flavors, increase the amount to compensate for the lack of salt. Bay leaves, fresh parsley, fresh dill, onions, and peppercorns give stock and soups flavor without added salt.

Celery, spinach, and various greens such as beets, collards, chard, and kale tend to be higher in sodium than most vegetables. Simmer them along with your other ingredients to help enhance the flavors.

Marinate poultry and fish for 24 hours with pepper, paprika, garlic, and onion powder. Wine, lemon juice, and flavored vinegars also help to accent the flavors of these meats. In some dishes, a little salt can make a big difference over the same dish with no salt.

A little Parmesan cheese or the use of one canned-with-salt ingredient is usually all that is needed.

TOPS AND BOTTOMS

The concept of "Tops and Bottoms" exemplifies a simple approach to good eating. Start with a "bottom," and add one or more "tops" to create a food encounter. This can be as simple as applesauce or stewed tomatoes served over a baked potato. Something more elaborate might be a corn tortilla topped with tomato slices and tuna salad, then heated through and finished off with a dollop of Garlic Yogurt Sauce.

SOME TOPS OPTIONS

Ragu or All Purpose Tomato Sauce
Steamed Fresh Vegetables
Fresh or frozen crushed berries
Canned pineapple
Ratatouille
Parmesan cheese
Low-fat cottage cheese plus herbs
Chopped onion
Onion powder
Fried onion

No oil dressings
Stir-fried vegetables
Gazpacho
Thick bean soups
Plain low-fat yogurt
Pesto sauce
Diced chicken or tuna
Canned tomatoes or
zucchini
Tabouli

SOME BOTTOMS OPTIONS

Pasta
Brown rice
Baked potato
Whole wheat pita bread
Corn tortilla (soft, not fried)
Bulgar
Millet
Beans

Cabbage
Sprouts
Brussel sprouts
Wild rice
Mashed potatoes
Squash
Greens, spinach
Mashed turnip

240

CLEAN CUISINE CHECKLIST

TOWARD POORER HEALTH

- [ ] DAILY FAST FOOD CONVENIENCE
- [ ] DAILY PACKAGED SNACKS
- [ ] DAILY FATTY DAIRIES
- [ ] DAILY FLESH

TOWARD BETTER HEALTH

- [ ] REFRIGERATOR/FREEZER/STOVE TOP/MICROWAVE
- [ ] SERVING-SIZE STORAGE CONTAINERS FOR RICE, PASTA, SOUPS.
- [ ] SERVING-SIZE TRANSPARENT STORAGE BAGS
- [ ] WEEKLY SHOPPING/COOKING/PLANNING TIMES
- [ ] "EQUATORIAL" ETHNIC TOP AND BOTTOM DISHES
- [ ] SHOP-THE-WALLS AT YOUR SUPERMARKET
- [ ] WATCH FOR EMERGING FAT-FREE ITEMS

241

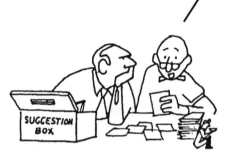

10 | EATING OUT ACTION STEPS

BROWN BAGGING IT

...A LITTLE ECCENTRICITY FOR HEALTH'S SAKE

He had begun brown-bagging his lunch several years ago. It was one of those small calculations required of everybody these days for that extra decade of survival. But he does brown-bag with a difference. In his desk he keeps silverware, a bowl, a placemat and napkins. "Everything but a flaming taper," a fellow worker once observed on his way out to lunch.

The man was a patient of mine I had persuaded to cut his meat intake in half. These days he lunches on, and at, his desk: Another patient, of more diamond hard habits, still eats out. He usually opts for a chopped sirloin called the Quick Fix. It's hamburger with presence, heavily garnished and with a supporting cast of French fries.

243

"A needed break in the day's routine," he explains. But from another point of view, it's yet another round lost in the struggle against cholesterol and calories. The typical fat-saturated lunch of hamburger and fries can exceed 800 calories.

An alternative lunch break, one that allows time for shopping, a committee meeting, a fitness walk or whatever, could consist of fruit and nuts - not dried fruit and nuts, they're for the trail - but two different pieces of fresh fruit and a palmful of walnuts. The lid of an 8-ounce jar makes a handy serving dish and portion-control device. Salt dependent individuals who are unable to go cold turkey can apply a pinch of their favorite seasoning from a shaker kept in their desk drawer.

The best nuts are those rich in polyunsaturates. This rules out coconut and other tropical nuts as their fats are saturated. A heart-supporting mix consists of equal parts peanuts, sunflower seeds and walnuts. Together with an apple and banana, they provide no more than 500 calories; a good serving of protein, vitamins and minerals; but for the weight prone, too much fat. Such a lunch is light enough that there's no post-prandial torpor and no mid afternoon sugar slim - all at great convenience and for less than a dollar.

Another at-the-desk refreshment for mid-morning or mid-afternoon breaks features vegetables: single serving canned vegetables. Granted, we're not talking mainstream munching here, but it makes more nutrition sense than the ubiquitous jellied donut - more protein, fiber, potassium and appetite control. And no fat.

Even canned, much food value remains in vegetables, and the convenience of keeping them almost indefinitely in a drawer made for the economy of no spoilage. So put aside the prune danish and try one of today's newest, low-salt, canned offerings from the food industry. There are asparagus tips, crunchy corn nibblets, or zucchini, or peas, or beans and so on. All are precooked for consumption at desktop temperature. All are low in fat and rich in fiber.

Brown bagging it is one way to protect yourself from luncheon excess, not to mention the 10 AM and 3 PM sugar hits.

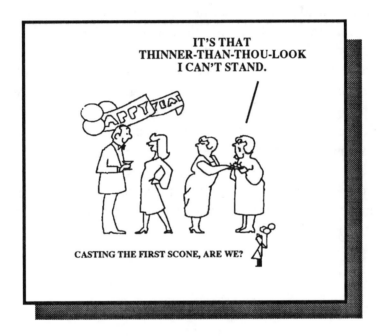

HANDLING HOLIDAYS ACTION STEPS

ABUNDANCE COMES ... AND STAYS

IN A CYCLE OF SEASONS

Jolly feeding pressures from family and friends at holiday times are not always the signs of affection and hospitality that they may seem. You are especially at risk if you have recently lost weight and the weight loss is noticeable. You are then a challenge to all those others who want to lose weight and haven't been successful. It's a challenge to be defeated, but often it's the host or hostess who wins when they cajole you into playing the good sport and agreeably sampling all the latest in holidays treats.

The smart slim, or slimming, guest will look upon parties and receptions as an opportunity to socialize, to renew friendships, to wheel and deal, to score points or, simply, score. The smart guest will circulate and share in everything but the feeding frenzy. He or she will be enjoying or surviving any festive event of the season of Too Much by prefeeding, nibbling and planning.

247

Prefeeding means arriving at a party neither hungry nor thirsty. Eat an apple or a banana before you set out, or a bowl of popcorn. Have a cup of tea or a diet pop or a glass of water. This allows the polite decline of "Thanks, I'm comfortable," to roll trippingly off the tongue when pressed by host, hostess or circulating tray-bearers.

Nibbling means small bites separated by long pauses and never finishing all that's offered, whether of finger food or sit down seven course dinners. Nibbling means looking for fruits and vegetables and avoiding meat, cheese and hot appetizers. (Hot appetizers would dry out if not evaporation-proofed by oil). Clean dips can be made with non-fat yogurt, non-fat cottage cheese, egg white, or thinned mashed potato, then given a fruit flavor with juice or pulp or a savory flavor with onion, garlic, lemon and horseradish. Even a bowl of sprinkle cheese such as Parmesan makes for a cleaner dip.

Planning involves knowing what you want and arranging to get there. Take a clean gift to the party - a fifth of non-alcohol wine or beer, wild mushrooms, gourmet flat bread, gourmet mustard, etc. Carry a non-fat topping (in a single serving packet) in purse or pocket. Planning also means allowing time to rest and recover from the drive.

HANDLING HOLIDAYS CHECKLIST

HEALTH UNDERMINING PARTY HABITS

- [ ] HOT APPETIZERS (ALWAYS FATTY)
- [ ] CHEESE CHUNKS / MYSTERY MEAT CHUNKS
- [ ] CHIPS / NUTS / PACKAGED SNACKS
- [ ] FATTY DIPS / SAUCES / CREAMS / DRESSINGS
- [ ] COLD CUTS / SAUSAGES / MYSTERY MEAT BALLS
- [ ] TOPPINGS / COATINGS / SPREADS / BREADINGS
- [ ] ALCOHOL DISSOLVES WILLPOWER / FIX YOUR OWN

HEALTH PROMOTING PARTY HABITS

- [ ] EAT BEFORE YOU GET THERE (APPLE / BANANA)
- [ ] CONVERSE WITH YOUR BACK TO THE FOOD
- [ ] SIP A NON-ALCOHOLIC DRINK / SPRITZER / JUICES
- [ ] LOOK FOR CHUNKED FRUIT OR VEGETABLE BITES
- [ ] LOOK FOR NON-FAT DIPS / DESSERTS / TOPPINGS
- [ ] EAT THE CENTERPIECE
- [ ] HAVE A NON-FAT SALAD OIL IN PURSE OR POCKET
- [ ] TAKE A NON-FAT DISH TO THE KITCHEN

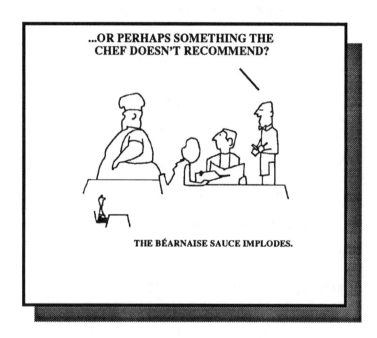

12 PROTEIN REASSURANCES

WHERE'S THE BEEF?

...YOU'LL BE SURPRISED

For several years after World War II the entire German population suffered food shortages. They ate a diet quite deficient by today's standards, deriving about 80% of their calories from flour and the remaining 20% from vegetables. There was no milk and no meat, except for a tiny weekly serving of fatty sausage. Yet to the surprise of nutritionists who later studied children who had grown up in those years, such a diet left no sign of physical or mental effects. Indeed, in a selected sub-set of children given dried milk supplements as a test of the potential contribution of milk to the "poor" diet, no extra growth or tissue benefits could be demonstrated.

251

Many cultures consume half as much protein as we do, indeed half our RDA(Recommended Daily Allowance) for protein, without apparent ill health. Our RDA for protein is an educated guess produced by nutrition scientists at the turn of the century, using young adult male manual laborers as their target population.

One widely used diet to help prevent heart attacks is the Pritikin diet, which severely restricts animal proteins. Yet it's actually a high protein diet. Nutrient analysis of its vegetables, grains and legumes reveal much protein. Indeed, five or six servings easily meet the day's protein needs.

A recent sign over a supermarket display of picnic hot dogs declared that each one provided as much protein as an egg. True. Ignored in the pitch however, is that only 35 of the dog's 145 calories, come from protein. The remaining 110, or a whopping 70% of its calories, come from fat.

THE PROTEIN CONTENT
OF SOME COMMON FOODS

FOOD ITEM	SERV. SIZE	APPROX PROTEIN CONTNT. IN GRAMS	FOOD ITEM	SERV. SIZE	APPROX PROTEIN CONTNT. IN GRAMS
ARTICHOKE	1	3	MILK, WHOLE	1C	8
ASPARAGUS	1C	4	MILK, SKIM	1C	10
BEANS, DRIED	1 C	10	OATMEAL	1C	10
BEEF, HAMBURGER	3 OZ	15	OKRA	1C	4
BEEF, HOT DOG	1	10			
BEEF COLD CUTS	1 OZ	3	NUTS	3 OZ	12
BROCCOLI	1C	4			
BREAD, WHOLE GR.	SLCE	3	PASTA	2 OZ	8
BREAD WHITE	SLCE	1. 5	PEANUT BUTTER	2 TBS	9
BREAD RYE	SLCE	2	PEAS	1C	9
			POTATO	1	5
CHEESE	3 OZ	15			
CORNFLAKES	1C	2	RAISINS	1C	6
			RICE, BROWN	1C	4
EGGS	2	12	RICE, WHITE	1C	3
EGG WHITES	4	12			
			SEEDS	3 OZ	12
FARINA CEREAL	1C	6	SOYBEANS	1C	20
			SPINACH , GREENS	1C	5
GREEN BEANS	1C	2	SQUASH	1C	5
ICE CREAM	1C	5	WHEAT GERM	2 TBS	8
LENTILS	1C	6	YOGURT	1C	8

NUTRITION AUTHORITIES RECOMMEND FOR ADULTS 50 - 75 GRAMS
OF PROTEIN PER DAY, ALTHOUGH CULTURES HAVE BEEN STUDIED
THAT EAT HALF THAT OVER A LIFETIME WITHOUT DEFICIENCY SIGNS.

PART FIVE

CONTRACT NEGOTIATIONS

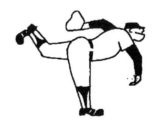

PRE-SEASON PLAY:
A 30 DAY GAME PLAN

Today's medical emergencies take years to happen, in fact about 20 to 30 years to the crisis, which then can happen in seconds. The chronic diseases which cripple and shorten our lives today, diseases such as heart disease, cancer and diabetes, are for the most part preventable and even reversible, provided that interventions are undertaken in time.

Such interventions must become habits, the most valuable health investments you can make. Habit change begins with a decision to lower some numbers - perhaps your weight, or blood pressure, or blood cholesterol.

Whatever your numbers, they reflect your daily habits. To change your numbers and your health prospects for the better, you must change your habits for the better, with fresh insights and information, which is what this book has been about. Now the time has come for the visionary adult in you to negotiate a contract with the child. Start slowly, you've got the rest of your life to get it all together. The next few pages provide an opportunity to set up 4 Weekly ScoreCards and a fresh Pre-Season 4 Week ScoreBoard. Play ball!

CONTRACT NEGOTIATIONS

YOUR STARTING ScoRECARD™

WEEK 1

1. RUNNING ALL THE BASES

SCORING: DAILY: 10   WEEKLY: 5   MONTHLY: 0
(MORE OR LESS)   (TWICE OR THRICE)   (SELDOM OR NEVER)

		SCORING	
		You	**Ideal**
	WHOLE FOOD HABITS		
FIRST BASE	FRESH / FROZEN / CANNED FRUITS:		10
	FRESH / FROZEN / CANNED VEGETABLES:		10
	WHOLE GRAIN BREADS / ROLLS / CEREALS / PASTAS:		10
	ADDITIONAL FIBER HABITS		
SECOND BASE	BEANS / PEAS / LENTILS:		10
	MUFFINS / BRANS / FIBERED CEREALS:		10
	FIBER SUPPLEMENTS-LAXATIVES / NUTS & SEEDS:		10
	LAXATION HABITS		
THIRD BASE	STOOLS: SOFT, FORMED & BUOYANT:		10
	PASSAGE: PAINLESS & BLOODLESS:		10
	AEROBIC FITNESS HABITS		
	BRISK WALKING, DANCING, RUNNING:		10
	TREADMILLING, AEROBICS, OTHER ACTIVITIES:		10
	RECREATION HABITS		
HOME PLATE	GARDENING, GOLFING, SWIMMING, OTHER:		10
	READING, HOBBYING, CONCERT-GOING, OTHER:		10

IF YOUR BASE-RUNNING IS:
ABOVE 100: FANTASTIC! KEEP IT UP
BETWEEN 75 AND 100:
   (YOU'RE ABOVE AVERAGE)   **Now add up
all the scores
from your habits.**
BELOW 50: YOU NEED A LITTLE R&R
   (REPAIR & RESTORATION)

YOUR BASE-RUNNING SCORE: 120

2. READING ALL THE PITCHES

(NOT ~~~~~~~)

WEEK 1

SCORING: **DAILY: 0**   **WEEKLY: 5**   **MONTHLY: 10**
(MORE OR LESS)   (TWICE OR THRICE)   (SELDOM OR NEVER)

		SCORING
FOOD FATS & OILS & CHOLESTEROL*		**You** / **Ideal**
GREASEBALL	BURGERS* / BACON-HAM* / FRANKS* / COLD CUTS*:	10
	% MILKS* / ICE CREAM* / CHEESE* / BUTTER*:	10
	DRESSINGS / MARG/MAYO* / FRIES° / PIZZA*/ RIBS*:	10
	CHIPS° / SNAX/ SWEET ROLLS / CAKE-PIE-COOKIES:	5
	BEEF-PORK-CHICKEN-TURKEY-FISH-SHRIMP*/ YOLK*	5
FOOD SALT SOURCES		
SALTY SLIDER	CANNED SOUPS/ COLD CEREALS/ PICKLES/ CHEESE:	5
	PKGED. DINNERS, DESSERTS, SNACKS*/ EATING OUT:	5
BIOSTRESS ISSUES		
BEANBALL	ANGRY : IRRITABLE-AGGRAVATED-TENSE:	5
	ANXIOUS : PRESSURED-DEADLINED-TENSE:	5
	BURNEDOUT: BORED-DISINTERESTED-DEPRESSED:	10
LIFESTYLE ISSUES		
	SICK DAYS-DRUGS-TABLETS-PILLS-ASPIRIN:	10
	LIQUOR-BEER-WINE-SMOKING / OTHER CHEMICALS:	10
FOOD-INDUCED ACHES, PAINS & CONGESTIONS		
SCREWBALL	HEAD : HEADACHES / SINUS /NASAL STUFFINESS:	10
	CHEST : TIGHTNESS / PHLEGM / WHEEZING-COUGH:	10
	ABDOMEN : ACHES / TENDERNESS / GAS / BLOATING:	10

*
* HIGH IN CHOLESTEROL
□ MAY CONTAIN CHOLESTEROL
   (BUTTER, EGG YOLK)
° MAY RAISE CHOLESTEROL
   (SAT. FATS, TRANS FATS)

YOUR PITCHES SCORE: 120
BASE RUNNING SCORE: 120
TOTAL PERFORMANCE 240

259

YOUR STARTING ScoreCard™

WEEK 2

1. RUNNING ALL THE BASES

SCORING: DAILY: 10   WEEKLY: 5   MONTHLY: 0
(MORE OR LESS) (TWICE OR THRICE) (SELDOM OR NEVER)

		SCORING You	Ideal
WHOLE FOOD HABITS			
FIRST BASE	FRESH / FROZEN / CANNED FRUITS:		10
	FRESH / FROZEN / CANNED VEGETABLES:		10
	WHOLE GRAIN BREADS / ROLLS / CEREALS / PASTAS:		10
ADDITIONAL FIBER HABITS			
SECOND BASE	BEANS / PEAS / LENTILS:		10
	MUFFINS / BRANS / FIBERED CEREALS:		10
	FIBER SUPPLEMENTS-LAXATIVES / NUTS & SEEDS:		10
LAXATION HABITS			
	STOOLS: SOFT, FORMED & BUOYANT:		10
	PASSAGE: PAINLESS & BLOODLESS:		10
AEROBIC FITNESS HABITS			
THIRD BASE	BRISK WALKING, DANCING, RUNNING:		10
	TREADMILLING, AEROBICS, OTHER ACTIVITIES:		10
RECREATION HABITS			
	GARDENING, GOLFING, SWIMMING, OTHER:		10
HOME PLATE	READING, HOBBYING, CONCERT-GOING, OTHER:		10

IF YOUR BASE-RUNNING IS:
ABOVE 100: FANTASTIC! KEEP IT UP
BETWEEN 75 AND 100:
(YOU'RE ABOVE AVERAGE)

BELOW 50: YOU NEED A LITTLE R&R
(REPAIR & RESTORATION)

Now add up all the scores from your habits.

YOUR BASE-RUNNING SCORE: | 120

WINNING THE WELLNESS GAME

2. READING ALL THE PITCHES

(NOT [ ])

WEEK 2

SCORING: DAILY: 0   WEEKLY: 5   MONTHLY: 10
(MORE OR LESS) (TWICE OR THRICE) (SELDOM OR NEVER)

SCORING
You | Ideal

FOOD FATS & OILS & CHOLESTEROL*		
GREASEBALL	BURGERS* / BACON-HAM* / FRANKS* / COLD CUTS*:	10
	% MILKS* / ICE CREAM* / CHEESE* / BUTTER*:	10
	DRESSINGS / MARG/MAYO* / FRIES / PIZZA*/ RIBS*:	10
	CHIPS / SNAX/ SWEET ROLLS / CAKE-PIE-COOKIES:	5
	BEEF-PORK-CHICKEN-TURKEY-FISH-SHRIMP*/ YOLK*	5
FOOD SALT SOURCES		
SALTY SLIDER	CANNED SOUPS/ COLD CEREALS/ PICKLES/ CHEESE:	5
	PKGED. DINNERS, DESSERTS, SNACKS*/ EATING OUT:	5
BIOSTRESS ISSUES		
BEANBALL	ANGRY : IRRITABLE-AGGRAVATED-TENSE:	5
	ANXIOUS : PRESSURED-DEADLINED-TENSE:	5
	BURNEDOUT: BORED-DISINTERESTED-DEPRESSED:	10
LIFESTYLE ISSUES		
	SICK DAYS-DRUGS-TABLETS-PILLS-ASPIRIN:	10
	LIQUOR-BEER-WINE-SMOKING / OTHER CHEMICALS:	10
FOOD-INDUCED ACHES, PAINS & CONGESTIONS		
SCREWBALL	HEAD : HEADACHES / SINUS /NASAL STUFFINESS:	10
	CHEST : TIGHTNESS / PHLEGM / WHEEZING-COUGH:	10
	ABDOMEN : ACHES / TENDERNESS / GAS / BLOATING:	10

*
* HIGH IN CHOLESTEROL
□ MAY CONTAIN CHOLESTEROL (BUTTER, EGG YOLK)
○ MAY RAISE CHOLESTEROL (SAT. FATS, TRANS FATS)

YOUR PITCHES SCORE: 120
BASE RUNNING SCORE: 120
TOTAL PERFORMANCE 240

COPYRIGHT © 1990 NATIONAL HEALTH SYSTEMS INC. ALL RIGHTS RESERVED

261

CONTRACT NEGOTIATIONS

WEEK 3

YOUR STARTING ScoReCARD™

1. RUNNING ALL THE BASES

SCORING: DAILY: 10   WEEKLY: 5   MONTHLY: 0
(MORE OR LESS) (TWICE OR THRICE) (SELDOM OR NEVER)

		SCORING	
		You	Ideal
WHOLE FOOD HABITS			
	FRESH / FROZEN / CANNED FRUITS:		10
	FRESH / FROZEN / CANNED VEGETABLES:		10
FIRST BASE	WHOLE GRAIN BREADS / ROLLS / CEREALS / PASTAS:		10
ADDITIONAL FIBER HABITS			
	BEANS / PEAS / LENTILS:		10
	MUFFINS / BRANS / FIBERED CEREALS:		10
SECOND BASE	FIBER SUPPLEMENTS-LAXATIVES / NUTS & SEEDS:		10
LAXATION HABITS			
	STOOLS: SOFT, FORMED & BUOYANT:		10
	PASSAGE: PAINLESS & BLOODLESS:		10
AEROBIC FITNESS HABITS			
	BRISK WALKING, DANCING, RUNNING:		10
THIRD BASE	TREADMILLING, AEROBICS, OTHER ACTIVITIES:		10
RECREATION HABITS			
	GARDENING, GOLFING, SWIMMING, OTHER:		10
HOME PLATE	READING, HOBBYING, CONCERT-GOING, OTHER:		10

IF YOUR BASE-RUNNING IS:
ABOVE 100: FANTASTIC! KEEP IT UP
BETWEEN 75 AND 100:
   (YOU'RE ABOVE AVERAGE)

BELOW 50: YOU NEED A LITTLE R&R
   (REPAIR & RESTORATION)

**Now add up
all the scores
from your habits.**

YOUR BASE-RUNNING SCORE: | 120

COPYRIGHT © 1990 NATIONAL HEALTH SYSTEMS INC. ALL RIGHTS RESERVED

2. READING ALL THE PITCHES

WEEK 3

(NOT ~~~~~~~~)

SCORING: DAILY: 0   WEEKLY: 5   MONTHLY: 10
(MORE OR LESS) (TWICE OR THRICE) (SELDOM OR NEVER)

		SCORING	
		You	Ideal
FOOD FATS & OILS & CHOLESTEROL*			
	BURGERS* / BACON-HAM* / FRANKS* / COLD CUTS*:		10
	% MILKS* / ICE CREAM* / CHEESE* / BUTTER*:		10
	DRESSINGS / MARG/MAYO* / FRIES° / PIZZA*/ RIBS*:		10
GREASEBALL	CHIPS° / SNAX/ SWEET ROLLS / CAKE-PIE-COOKIES:		5
	BEEF-PORK-CHICKEN-TURKEY-FISH-SHRIMP*/ YOLK*		5
FOOD SALT SOURCES			
	CANNED SOUPS/ COLD CEREALS/ PICKLES/ CHEESE:		5
SALTY SLIDER	PKGED. DINNERS, DESSERTS, SNACKS*/ EATING OUT:		5
BIOSTRESS ISSUES			
	ANGRY : IRRITABLE-AGGRAVATED-TENSE:		5
	ANXIOUS : PRESSURED-DEADLINED-TENSE:		5
	BURNEDOUT: BORED-DISINTERESTED-DEPRESSED:		10
LIFESTYLE ISSUES			
BEANBALL	SICK DAYS-DRUGS-TABLETS-PILLS-ASPIRIN:		10
	LIQUOR-BEER-WINE-SMOKING / OTHER CHEMICALS:		10
FOOD-INDUCED ACHES, PAINS & CONGESTIONS			
	HEAD : HEADACHES / SINUS /NASAL STUFFINESS:		10
	CHEST : TIGHTNESS / PHLEGM / WHEEZING-COUGH:		10
SCREWBALL	ABDOMEN : ACHES / TENDERNESS / GAS / BLOATING:		10

*
* HIGH IN CHOLESTEROL
□ MAY CONTAIN CHOLESTEROL
   (BUTTER, EGG YOLK)
° MAY RAISE CHOLESTEROL
   (SAT. FATS, TRANS FATS)

YOUR PITCHES SCORE:	120
BASE RUNNING SCORE:	120
TOTAL PERFORMANCE	240

CONTRACT NEGOTIATIONS

YOUR STARTING ScoReCARD™

WEEK 4

1. RUNNING ALL THE BASES

SCORING: DAILY: 10   WEEKLY: 5   MONTHLY: 0
(MORE OR LESS)   (TWICE OR THRICE)   (SELDOM OR NEVER)

		SCORING You	Ideal
WHOLE FOOD HABITS			
FIRST BASE	FRESH / FROZEN / CANNED FRUITS:		10
	FRESH / FROZEN / CANNED VEGETABLES:		10
	WHOLE GRAIN BREADS / ROLLS / CEREALS / PASTAS:		10
ADDITIONAL FIBER HABITS			
SECOND BASE	BEANS / PEAS / LENTILS:		10
	MUFFINS / BRANS / FIBERED CEREALS:		10
	FIBER SUPPLEMENTS-LAXATIVES / NUTS & SEEDS:		10
LAXATION HABITS			
	STOOLS: SOFT, FORMED & BUOYANT:		10
	PASSAGE: PAINLESS & BLOODLESS:		10
AEROBIC FITNESS HABITS			
THIRD BASE	BRISK WALKING, DANCING, RUNNING:		10
	TREADMILLING, AEROBICS, OTHER ACTIVITIES:		10
RECREATION HABITS			
HOME PLATE	GARDENING, GOLFING, SWIMMING, OTHER:		10
	READING, HOBBYING, CONCERT-GOING, OTHER:		10

IF YOUR BASE-RUNNING IS:
ABOVE 100: FANTASTIC! KEEP IT UP
BETWEEN 75 AND 100:
(YOU'RE ABOVE AVERAGE)
BELOW 50: YOU NEED A LITTLE R&R
(REPAIR & RESTORATION)

Now add up all the scores from your habits.

YOUR BASE-RUNNING SCORE: 120

2. READING ALL THE PITCHES

WEEK 4

(NOT _____)

SCORING: DAILY: 0   WEEKLY: 5   MONTHLY: 10
(MORE OR LESS)   (TWICE OR THRICE)   (SELDOM OR NEVER)

SCORING

		You	Ideal
FOOD FATS & OILS & CHOLESTEROL*			
	BURGERS* / BACON-HAM* / FRANKS* / COLD CUTS*:		10
	% MILKS* / ICE CREAM* / CHEESE* / BUTTER*:		10
	DRESSINGS° / MARG/MAYO* / FRIES° / PIZZA* / RIBS*:		10
GREASEBALL	CHIPS° / SNAX / SWEET ROLLS / CAKE-PIE-COOKIES°□:		5
	BEEF-PORK-CHICKEN-TURKEY-FISH-SHRIMP* / YOLK*		5
FOOD SALT SOURCES			
	CANNED SOUPS / COLD CEREALS / PICKLES / CHEESE:		5
SALTY SLIDER	PKGED. DINNERS, DESSERTS, SNACKS*°□ / EATING OUT°□:		5
BIOSTRESS ISSUES			
	ANGRY : IRRITABLE-AGGRAVATED-TENSE:		5
	ANXIOUS : PRESSURED-DEADLINED-TENSE:		5
	BURNEDOUT: BORED-DISINTERESTED-DEPRESSED:		10
LIFESTYLE ISSUES			
BEANBALL	SICK DAYS-DRUGS-TABLETS-PILLS-ASPIRIN:		10
	LIQUOR-BEER-WINE-SMOKING / OTHER CHEMICALS:		10
FOOD-INDUCED ACHES , PAINS & CONGESTIONS			
	HEAD : HEADACHES / SINUS /NASAL STUFFINESS:		10
	CHEST : TIGHTNESS / PHLEGM / WHEEZING-COUGH:		10
SCREWBALL	ABDOMEN : ACHES / TENDERNESS / GAS / BLOATING:		10

*
* HIGH IN CHOLESTEROL
□ MAY CONTAIN CHOLESTEROL
  (BUTTER, EGG YOLK)
° MAY RAISE CHOLESTEROL
  (SAT. FATS, TRANS FATS)

YOUR PITCHES SCORE: 120
BASE RUNNING SCORE: 120
TOTAL PERFORMANCE 240

COACH'S CORNER

A WORD ABOUT THE FITNESS MINUTE

The *Fitness Minute* can be an important strategy for weight control. It involves the use of a fitness activity and the calories expended in a minute to balance out extra calories taken on as special treats. *A Fitness Minute* is any activity that takes your warmed-up heart rate to 100-120 beats a minute, without discomfort, and holds it there for one minute. It could be an effort such as scrubbing floors and other chores; running, jumping, and bicycle pumping; being in the swim or at the gym; even dancing, prancing or heavy romancing.

The neat mathematics about a *Fitness Minute* is that it burns 10 calories. By dividing the calories of any food item, such as double-dip ice cream cone, by 10, you can automatically translate its calories into its cost.

A double-dip ice cream cone providing 300 calories would require 30 minutes of a fitness activity to erase those calories. A large apple providing 80 calories is completely burnt up by 8 minutes of fitness activity.

In summary, there are two budgets of consequence for the weight prone: dollars and *Fitness Minutes*.. And *both* budgets must be balanced.

WINNING THE WELLNESS GAME

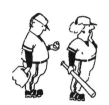

WINNING THE WELLNESS GAME

YOUR PRESEASON
ScoreBoard™

THE   ROOKIES

YOUR FIRST AT- BATS IN THE GAME

SCORE SCALE 300	YOUR SCORE TODAY	AFTER ONE WEEK	AFTER TWO WEEKS	AFTER THREE WEEKS	AFTER FOUR WEEKS	SYMBOLS
260						**CHOLESTROL** © Fasting blood cholesterol well under 200 is ideal
240						
210						
200						**BODYWEIGHT** Ⓦ Enter today's weight
190						
180						**BLD. PRESSR** Ⓟ Systolic blood pressure under 120 mm Hg is ideal
170						
160						**TOTAL SCORE** Ⓣ The global view of your progress. Above 200 ideal.
150						
140						
130						**BLOOD SUGR** Ⓢ Fasting blood sugar under 90 is ideal
120						
110						**HEART RATE** Ⓗ A resting heart rate under 60 beats per minute is ideal
100						
90						
80						**NEXT MONTH:** (USING SYMBOLS) ENTER TODAY'S SCORE IN SCORE SCALE COLUMN OF SEASON'S PLAY ScoreCard
70						
60						
50						

IT'S ALL ABOUT NUMBERS. GET TO KNOW THE WELLNESS RANGE.

IN SEASON PLAY:
A SIX-MONTH GAME PLAN

Getting there and staying there ... the two most important elements of any wellness effort; and effort it is, at least in its early stages. Your first month has probably provided lots of personal evidence in support of this experience.

Now it's time to make a longer deal with yourself; to sign on for a season of play by making a contract with 5 specific elements:

1) It's Specific: the ScoreCard pinpoints
                           items for change.

2) It's Measurable: the ScoreCard logs
                           frequencies.

3) It's Agreed upon: the texts of Parts II and III
                           provide reasons to review.

4) It's Rewarding: like feeling and looking
                           better.

5) It's Trackable: the ScoreBoard's all about
                           tracking performance.

SMART is the contract's acronym and SMART is the individual with the foresight to put it into play. Have a look at the entry items in the contract on the next page and sign on for a good season.

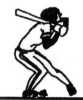

A 6 MONTH PERSONAL GAME PLAN

1   These really apply to me:
_____
_____
_____
_____

2   I've got to stop:
_____
_____
_____
_____

3   I've got to start:
_____
_____
_____
_____

4   I'll feel these improvements:
_____
_____
_____
_____

5   I'll be able to measure this:
_____

WINNING THE WELLNESS GAME
YOUR SEASON'S PLAY
ScoreBoard™

THE   PROS

SCORE SCALE	FIRST MONTH	SECOND MONTH	THIRD MONTH	FOURTH MONTH	FIFTH MONTH	SIXTH MONTH
450 +						
400						
350						
300						
290						
280						
270						
260						
250						
240						
230						Ⓣ
220						
210						
200						
190						
180						
170						
160						Ⓒ
150						
140						
130						
120						
110						Ⓟ
100						
90						
80						Ⓢ
70						
60						
50	ENTER YOUR					Ⓗ
40	SYMBOLS & NUMBERS HERE					SYMBOLS SUGGEST IDEAL LEVELS

271

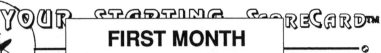

YOUR STARTING ScoreCard™

FIRST MONTH

1. RUNNING ALL THE BASES

SCORING: DAILY: 10   WEEKLY: 5   MONTHLY: 0
(MORE OR LESS) (TWICE OR THRICE) (SELDOM OR NEVER)

		SCORING You	Ideal
WHOLE FOOD HABITS			
FIRST BASE	FRESH / FROZEN / CANNED FRUITS:		10
	FRESH / FROZEN / CANNED VEGETABLES:		10
	WHOLE GRAIN BREADS / ROLLS / CEREALS / PASTAS:		10
ADDITIONAL FIBER HABITS			
SECOND BASE	BEANS / PEAS / LENTILS:		10
	MUFFINS / BRANS / FIBERED CEREALS:		10
	FIBER SUPPLEMENTS-LAXATIVES / NUTS & SEEDS:		10
LAXATION HABITS			
THIRD BASE	STOOLS: SOFT, FORMED & BUOYANT:		10
	PASSAGE: PAINLESS & BLOODLESS:		10
AEROBIC FITNESS HABITS			
	BRISK WALKING, DANCING, RUNNING:		10
	TREADMILLING, AEROBICS, OTHER ACTIVITIES:		10
RECREATION HABITS			
HOME PLATE	GARDENING, GOLFING, SWIMMING, OTHER:		10
	READING, HOBBYING, CONCERT-GOING, OTHER:		10

IF YOUR BASE-RUNNING IS:
ABOVE 100: FANTASTIC! KEEP IT UP
BETWEEN 75 AND 100:
(YOU'RE ABOVE AVERAGE)

BELOW 50: YOU NEED A LITTLE R&R
(REPAIR & RESTORATION)

Now add up all the scores from your habits.

YOUR BASE-RUNNING SCORE: | 120

2. READING ALL THE PITCHES

(NOT ~~~~~~~~~~~~~~~)

FIRST MONTH

SCORING: DAILY: 0   WEEKLY: 5   MONTHLY: 10
(MORE OR LESS)   (TWICE OR THRICE)   (SELDOM OR NEVER)

		SCORING
		You / **Ideal**
FOOD FATS & OILS & CHOLESTEROL*		
GREASEBALL	BURGERS* / BACON-HAM* / FRANKS* / COLD CUTS*:	10
	% MILKS* / ICE CREAM* / CHEESE* / BUTTER*:	10
	DRESSINGS / MARG/MAYO* / FRIES° / PIZZA*/ RIBS*:	10
	CHIPS° / SNAX/ SWEET ROLLS / CAKE-PIE-COOKIES°□:	5
	BEEF-PORK-CHICKEN-TURKEY-FISH-SHRIMP*/ YOLK*	5
FOOD SALT SOURCES		
SALTY SLIDER	CANNED SOUPS/ COLD CEREALS/ PICKLES/ CHEESE:	5
	PKGED. DINNERS, DESSERTS, SNACKS*/ EATING OUT:	5
BIOSTRESS ISSUES		
BEANBALL	ANGRY : IRRITABLE-AGGRAVATED-TENSE:	5
	ANXIOUS : PRESSURED-DEADLINED-TENSE:	5
	BURNEDOUT: BORED-DISINTERESTED-DEPRESSED:	10
LIFESTYLE ISSUES		
	SICK DAYS-DRUGS-TABLETS-PILLS-ASPIRIN:	10
	LIQUOR-BEER-WINE-SMOKING / OTHER CHEMICALS:	10
FOOD-INDUCED ACHES, PAINS & CONGESTIONS		
SCREWBALL	HEAD : HEADACHES / SINUS /NASAL STUFFINESS:	10
	CHEST : TIGHTNESS / PHLEGM / WHEEZING-COUGH:	10
	ABDOMEN : ACHES / TENDERNESS / GAS / BLOATING:	10

* HIGH IN CHOLESTEROL
□ MAY CONTAIN CHOLESTEROL
   (BUTTER, EGG YOLK)
° MAY RAISE CHOLESTEROL
   (SAT. FATS, TRANS FATS)

YOUR PITCHES SCORE: | 120
BASE RUNNING SCORE: | 120
TOTAL PERFORMANCE | 240

273

CONTRACT NEGOTIATIONS

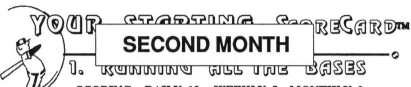

YOUR STARTING ScoreCard™

SECOND MONTH

1. RUNNING ALL THE BASES

SCORING: DAILY: 10   WEEKLY: 5   MONTHLY: 0
(MORE OR LESS) (TWICE OR THRICE) (SELDOM OR NEVER)

		SCORING	
	WHOLE FOOD HABITS	**You**	**Ideal**
FIRST BASE	FRESH / FROZEN / CANNED FRUITS:		10
	FRESH / FROZEN / CANNED VEGETABLES:		10
	WHOLE GRAIN BREADS / ROLLS / CEREALS / PASTAS:		10
	ADDITIONAL FIBER HABITS		
SECOND BASE	BEANS / PEAS / LENTILS:		10
	MUFFINS / BRANS / FIBERED CEREALS:		10
	FIBER SUPPLEMENTS-LAXATIVES / NUTS & SEEDS:		10
	LAXATION HABITS		
THIRD BASE	STOOLS: SOFT, FORMED & BUOYANT:		10
	PASSAGE: PAINLESS & BLOODLESS:		10
	AEROBIC FITNESS HABITS		
	BRISK WALKING, DANCING, RUNNING:		10
	TREADMILLING, AEROBICS, OTHER ACTIVITIES:		10
HOME PLATE	**RECREATION HABITS**		
	GARDENING, GOLFING, SWIMMING, OTHER:		10
	READING, HOBBYING, CONCERT-GOING, OTHER:		10

IF YOUR BASE-RUNNING IS:
ABOVE 100: FANTASTIC! KEEP IT UP
BETWEEN 75 AND 100:
(YOU'RE ABOVE AVERAGE)

BELOW 50: YOU NEED A LITTLE R&R
(REPAIR & RESTORATION)

**Now add up
all the scores
from your habits.**

YOUR BASE-RUNNING SCORE: | 120

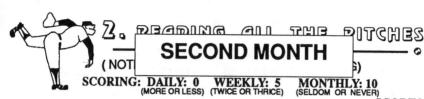

2. READING ALL THE PITCHES
(NOT ~~~~~~~~~~~)

SECOND MONTH

SCORING: **DAILY: 0** **WEEKLY: 5** **MONTHLY: 10**
(MORE OR LESS) (TWICE OR THRICE) (SELDOM OR NEVER)

		SCORING	
		You	Ideal
FOOD FATS & OILS & CHOLESTEROL*			
	BURGERS* / BACON-HAM* / FRANKS* / COLD CUTS*:		10
	% MILKS* / ICE CREAM* / CHEESE* / BUTTER*:		10
	DRESSINGS / MARG/MAYO* / FRIES° / PIZZA*/ RIBS*:		10
GREASEBALL	CHIPS° / SNAX/ SWEET ROLLS / CAKE-PIE-COOKIES:		5
	BEEF-PORK-CHICKEN-TURKEY-FISH-SHRIMP*/ YOLK*		5
FOOD SALT SOURCES			
	CANNED SOUPS/ COLD CEREALS/ PICKLES/ CHEESE:		5
SALTY SLIDER	PKGED. DINNERS, DESSERTS, SNACKS*/ EATING OUT:		5
BIOSTRESS ISSUES			
	ANGRY : IRRITABLE-AGGRAVATED-TENSE:		5
	ANXIOUS : PRESSURED-DEADLINED-TENSE:		5
	BURNEDOUT: BORED-DISINTERESTED-DEPRESSED:		10
LIFESTYLE ISSUES			
	SICK DAYS-DRUGS-TABLETS-PILLS-ASPIRIN:		10
BEANBALL	LIQUOR-BEER-WINE-SMOKING / OTHER CHEMICALS:		10
FOOD-INDUCED ACHES, PAINS & CONGESTIONS			
	HEAD : HEADACHES / SINUS /NASAL STUFFINESS:		10
	CHEST : TIGHTNESS / PHLEGM / WHEEZING-COUGH:		10
SCREWBALL	ABDOMEN : ACHES / TENDERNESS / GAS / BLOATING:		10

*
* HIGH IN CHOLESTEROL
□ MAY CONTAIN CHOLESTEROL
    (BUTTER, EGG YOLK)
° MAY RAISE CHOLESTEROL
    (SAT. FATS, TRANS FATS)

YOUR PITCHES SCORE: 120
BASE RUNNING SCORE: 120
TOTAL PERFORMANCE 240

CONTRACT NEGOTIATIONS

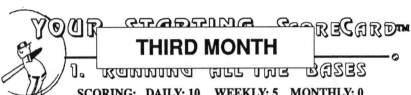

YOUR STARTING ScoRECARD™

THIRD MONTH

1. RUNNING ALL THE BASES

SCORING: DAILY: 10   WEEKLY: 5   MONTHLY: 0
(MORE OR LESS) (TWICE OR THRICE) (SELDOM OR NEVER)

		SCORING	
		You	Ideal
	WHOLE FOOD HABITS		
FIRST BASE	FRESH / FROZEN / CANNED FRUITS:		10
	FRESH / FROZEN / CANNED VEGETABLES:		10
	WHOLE GRAIN BREADS / ROLLS / CEREALS / PASTAS:		10
	ADDITIONAL FIBER HABITS		
SECOND BASE	BEANS / PEAS / LENTILS:		10
	MUFFINS / BRANS / FIBERED CEREALS:		10
	FIBER SUPPLEMENTS-LAXATIVES / NUTS & SEEDS:		10
	LAXATION HABITS		
THIRD BASE	STOOLS: SOFT, FORMED & BUOYANT:		10
	PASSAGE: PAINLESS & BLOODLESS:		10
	AEROBIC FITNESS HABITS		
	BRISK WALKING, DANCING, RUNNING:		10
	TREADMILLING, AEROBICS, OTHER ACTIVITIES:		10
	RECREATION HABITS		
HOME PLATE	GARDENING, GOLFING, SWIMMING, OTHER:		10
	READING, HOBBYING, CONCERT-GOING, OTHER:		10

IF YOUR BASE-RUNNING IS:
ABOVE 100: FANTASTIC! KEEP IT UP
BETWEEN 75 AND 100:
    (YOU'RE ABOVE AVERAGE)

BELOW 50: YOU NEED A LITTLE R&R
    (REPAIR & RESTORATION)

**Now add up
all the scores
from your habits.**

YOUR BASE-RUNNING SCORE:	120

2. READING ALL THE PITCHES

THIRD MONTH

(NOT ~~~~~~~~~~~~)

SCORING: DAILY: 0   WEEKLY: 5   MONTHLY: 10
(MORE OR LESS)   (TWICE OR THRICE)   (SELDOM OR NEVER)

SCORING

FOOD FATS & OILS & CHOLESTEROL*		You	Ideal
GREASEBALL	BURGERS* / BACON-HAM* / FRANKS* / COLD CUTS*:		10
	% MILKS* / ICE CREAM* / CHEESE* / BUTTER*:		10
	DRESSINGS / MARG/MAYO* / FRIES / PIZZA* / RIBS*:		10
	CHIPS / SNAX/ SWEET ROLLS / CAKE-PIE-COOKIES:		5
	BEEF-PORK-CHICKEN-TURKEY-FISH-SHRIMP* / YOLK*		5
FOOD SALT SOURCES			
SALTY SLIDER	CANNED SOUPS/ COLD CEREALS/ PICKLES/ CHEESE:		5
	PKGED. DINNERS, DESSERTS, SNACKS* / EATING OUT:		5
BIOSTRESS ISSUES			
BEANBALL	ANGRY : IRRITABLE-AGGRAVATED-TENSE:		5
	ANXIOUS : PRESSURED-DEADLINED-TENSE:		5
	BURNEDOUT: BORED-DISINTERESTED-DEPRESSED:		10
LIFESTYLE ISSUES			
	SICK DAYS-DRUGS-TABLETS-PILLS-ASPIRIN:		10
	LIQUOR-BEER-WINE-SMOKING / OTHER CHEMICALS:		10
FOOD-INDUCED ACHES, PAINS & CONGESTIONS			
SCREWBALL	HEAD : HEADACHES / SINUS /NASAL STUFFINESS:		10
	CHEST : TIGHTNESS / PHLEGM / WHEEZING-COUGH:		10
	ABDOMEN : ACHES / TENDERNESS / GAS / BLOATING:		10

* • HIGH IN CHOLESTEROL
□ MAY CONTAIN CHOLESTEROL
(BUTTER, EGG YOLK)
○ MAY RAISE CHOLESTEROL
(SAT. FATS, TRANS FATS)

YOUR PITCHES SCORE:	120
BASE RUNNING SCORE:	120
TOTAL PERFORMANCE	240

277

CONTRACT NEGOTIATIONS

YOUR STARTING ScoreCARD™
FOURTH MONTH
1. RUNNING ALL THE BASES

SCORING: DAILY: 10   WEEKLY: 5   MONTHLY: 0
(MORE OR LESS) (TWICE OR THRICE) (SELDOM OR NEVER)

		SCORING You	Ideal
WHOLE FOOD HABITS			
FIRST BASE	FRESH / FROZEN / CANNED FRUITS:		10
	FRESH / FROZEN / CANNED VEGETABLES:		10
	WHOLE GRAIN BREADS / ROLLS / CEREALS / PASTAS:		10
ADDITIONAL FIBER HABITS			
SECOND BASE	BEANS / PEAS / LENTILS:		10
	MUFFINS / BRANS / FIBERED CEREALS:		10
	FIBER SUPPLEMENTS-LAXATIVES / NUTS & SEEDS:		10
LAXATION HABITS			
THIRD BASE	STOOLS: SOFT, FORMED & BUOYANT:		10
	PASSAGE: PAINLESS & BLOODLESS:		10
AEROBIC FITNESS HABITS			
	BRISK WALKING, DANCING, RUNNING:		10
	TREADMILLING, AEROBICS, OTHER ACTIVITIES:		10
RECREATION HABITS			
HOME PLATE	GARDENING, GOLFING, SWIMMING, OTHER:		10
	READING, HOBBYING, CONCERT-GOING, OTHER:		10

IF YOUR BASE-RUNNING IS:
ABOVE 100: FANTASTIC! KEEP IT UP
BETWEEN 75 AND 100:
(YOU'RE ABOVE AVERAGE)
BELOW 50: YOU NEED A LITTLE R&R
(REPAIR & RESTORATION)

Now add up all the scores from your habits.

YOUR BASE-RUNNING SCORE: | 120

2. READING ALL THE PITCHES

FOURTH MONTH

(NOT   )

SCORING: DAILY: 0   WEEKLY: 5   MONTHLY: 10
(MORE OR LESS)   (TWICE OR THRICE)   (SELDOM OR NEVER)

		SCORING
		You Ideal
FOOD FATS & OILS & CHOLESTEROL*		
GREASEBALL	BURGERS* / BACON-HAM* / FRANKS* / COLD CUTS*:	10
	% MILKS* / ICE CREAM* / CHEESE* / BUTTER*:	10
	DRESSINGS / MARG/MAYO* / FRIES / PIZZA*/ RIBS*:	10
	CHIPS / SNAX/ SWEET ROLLS / CAKE-PIE-COOKIES:	5
	BEEF-PORK-CHICKEN-TURKEY-FISH-SHRIMP*/ YOLK*	5
FOOD SALT SOURCES		
SALTY SLIDER	CANNED SOUPS/ COLD CEREALS/ PICKLES/ CHEESE:	5
	PKGED. DINNERS, DESSERTS, SNACKS*/ EATING OUT:	5
BIOSTRESS ISSUES		
BEANBALL	ANGRY : IRRITABLE-AGGRAVATED-TENSE:	5
	ANXIOUS : PRESSURED-DEADLINED-TENSE:	5
	BURNEDOUT: BORED-DISINTERESTED-DEPRESSED:	10
LIFESTYLE ISSUES		
	SICK DAYS-DRUGS-TABLETS-PILLS-ASPIRIN:	10
	LIQUOR-BEER-WINE-SMOKING / OTHER CHEMICALS:	10
FOOD-INDUCED ACHES, PAINS & CONGESTIONS		
SCREWBALL	HEAD : HEADACHES / SINUS /NASAL STUFFINESS:	10
	CHEST : TIGHTNESS / PHLEGM / WHEEZING-COUGH:	10
	ABDOMEN : ACHES / TENDERNESS / GAS / BLOATING:	10

*
* HIGH IN CHOLESTEROL
□ MAY CONTAIN CHOLESTEROL (BUTTER, EGG YOLK)
○ MAY RAISE CHOLESTEROL (SAT. FATS, TRANS FATS)

YOUR PITCHES SCORE:	120
BASE RUNNING SCORE:	120
TOTAL PERFORMANCE	240

YOUR STARTING ScoreCard™

FIFTH MONTH

1. RUNNING ALL THE BASES

SCORING: DAILY: 10   WEEKLY: 5   MONTHLY: 0
(MORE OR LESS) (TWICE OR THRICE) (SELDOM OR NEVER)

		SCORING You Ideal
WHOLE FOOD HABITS		
FIRST BASE	FRESH / FROZEN / CANNED FRUITS:	10
	FRESH / FROZEN / CANNED VEGETABLES:	10
	WHOLE GRAIN BREADS / ROLLS / CEREALS / PASTAS:	10
ADDITIONAL FIBER HABITS		
SECOND BASE	BEANS / PEAS / LENTILS:	10
	MUFFINS / BRANS / FIBERED CEREALS:	10
	FIBER SUPPLEMENTS-LAXATIVES / NUTS & SEEDS:	10
LAXATION HABITS		
THIRD BASE	STOOLS: SOFT, FORMED & BUOYANT:	10
	PASSAGE: PAINLESS & BLOODLESS:	10
AEROBIC FITNESS HABITS		
	BRISK WALKING, DANCING, RUNNING:	10
	TREADMILLING, AEROBICS, OTHER ACTIVITIES:	10
RECREATION HABITS		
HOME PLATE	GARDENING, GOLFING, SWIMMING, OTHER:	10
	READING, HOBBYING, CONCERT-GOING, OTHER:	10

IF YOUR BASE-RUNNING IS:
ABOVE 100: FANTASTIC! KEEP IT UP
BETWEEN 75 AND 100:
    (YOU'RE ABOVE AVERAGE)

BELOW 50: YOU NEED A LITTLE R&R
    (REPAIR & RESTORATION)

Now add up all the scores from your habits.

YOUR BASE-RUNNING SCORE: | 120

2. READING ALL THE PITCHES
(NOT   )

FIFTH MONTH

SCORING: DAILY: 0 (MORE OR LESS)   **WEEKLY: 5** (TWICE OR THRICE)   **MONTHLY: 10** (SELDOM OR NEVER)

FOOD FATS & OILS & CHOLESTEROL*	You	Ideal
BURGERS* / BACON-HAM* / FRANKS* / COLD CUTS*:		10
% MILKS* / ICE CREAM* / CHEESE* / BUTTER*:		10
DRESSINGS / MARG/MAYO* / FRIES / PIZZA*/ RIBS*:		10
CHIPS / SNAX/ SWEET ROLLS / CAKE-PIE-COOKIES:		5
BEEF-PORK-CHICKEN-TURKEY-FISH-SHRIMP*/ YOLK*		5
FOOD SALT SOURCES		
CANNED SOUPS/ COLD CEREALS/ PICKLES/ CHEESE:		5
PKGED. DINNERS, DESSERTS, SNACKS*/ EATING OUT:		5
BIOSTRESS ISSUES		
ANGRY : IRRITABLE-AGGRAVATED-TENSE:		5
ANXIOUS : PRESSURED-DEADLINED-TENSE:		5
BURNEDOUT: BORED-DISINTERESTED-DEPRESSED:		10
LIFESTYLE ISSUES		
SICK DAYS-DRUGS-TABLETS-PILLS-ASPIRIN:		10
LIQUOR-BEER-WINE-SMOKING / OTHER CHEMICALS:		10
FOOD-INDUCED ACHES, PAINS & CONGESTIONS		
HEAD : HEADACHES / SINUS /NASAL STUFFINESS:		10
CHEST : TIGHTNESS / PHLEGM / WHEEZING-COUGH:		10
ABDOMEN : ACHES / TENDERNESS / GAS / BLOATING:		10

GREASEBALL · SALTY SLIDER · BEANBALL · SCREWBALL

* · HIGH IN CHOLESTEROL
□ MAY CONTAIN CHOLESTEROL (BUTTER, EGG YOLK)
○ MAY RAISE CHOLESTEROL (SAT. FATS, TRANS FATS)

YOUR PITCHES SCORE: 120
BASE RUNNING SCORE: 120
TOTAL PERFORMANCE 240

281

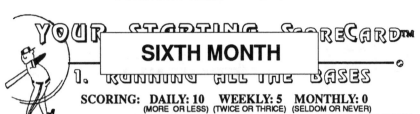

SIXTH MONTH

1. RUNNING ALL THE BASES

SCORING: DAILY: 10   WEEKLY: 5   MONTHLY: 0
(MORE OR LESS) (TWICE OR THRICE) (SELDOM OR NEVER)

		SCORING	
		You	Ideal
	WHOLE FOOD HABITS		
FIRST BASE	FRESH / FROZEN / CANNED FRUITS:		10
	FRESH / FROZEN / CANNED VEGETABLES:		10
	WHOLE GRAIN BREADS / ROLLS / CEREALS / PASTAS:		10
	ADDITIONAL FIBER HABITS		
SECOND BASE	BEANS / PEAS / LENTILS:		10
	MUFFINS / BRANS / FIBERED CEREALS:		10
	FIBER SUPPLEMENTS-LAXATIVES / NUTS & SEEDS:		10
	LAXATION HABITS		
THIRD BASE	STOOLS: SOFT, FORMED & BUOYANT:		10
	PASSAGE: PAINLESS & BLOODLESS:		10
	AEROBIC FITNESS HABITS		
	BRISK WALKING, DANCING, RUNNING:		10
	TREADMILLING, AEROBICS, OTHER ACTIVITIES:		10
	RECREATION HABITS		
HOME PLATE	GARDENING, GOLFING, SWIMMING, OTHER:		10
	READING, HOBBYING, CONCERT-GOING, OTHER:		10

IF YOUR BASE-RUNNING IS:
ABOVE 100: FANTASTIC! KEEP IT UP
BETWEEN 75 AND 100:
    (YOU'RE ABOVE AVERAGE)

BELOW 50: YOU NEED A LITTLE R&R
    (REPAIR & RESTORATION)

**Now add up
all the scores
from your habits.**

YOUR BASE-RUNNING SCORE: 120

2. READING ALL THE PITCHES

SIXTH MONTH

(NOT)

SCORING: DAILY: 0 (MORE OR LESS)   **WEEKLY: 5** (TWICE OR THRICE)   **MONTHLY: 10** (SELDOM OR NEVER)

FOOD FATS & OILS & CHOLESTEROL*	SCORING You	Ideal
BURGERS* / BACON-HAM* / FRANKS* / COLD CUTS*:		10
% MILKS* / ICE CREAM* / CHEESE* / BUTTER*:		10
DRESSINGS / MARG/MAYO* / FRIES° / PIZZA*/ RIBS*:		10
CHIPS° / SNAX/ SWEET ROLLS / CAKE-PIE-COOKIES°□:		5
BEEF-PORK-CHICKEN-TURKEY-FISH-SHRIMP*/ YOLK*		5
FOOD SALT SOURCES		
CANNED SOUPS/ COLD CEREALS/ PICKLES/ CHEESE:		5
PKGED. DINNERS, DESSERTS, SNACKS*/ EATING OUT°□:		5
BIOSTRESS ISSUES		
ANGRY : IRRITABLE-AGGRAVATED-TENSE:		5
ANXIOUS : PRESSURED-DEADLINED-TENSE:		5
BURNEDOUT: BORED-DISINTERESTED-DEPRESSED:		10
LIFESTYLE ISSUES		
SICK DAYS-DRUGS-TABLETS-PILLS-ASPIRIN:		10
LIQUOR-BEER-WINE-SMOKING / OTHER CHEMICALS:		10
FOOD-INDUCED ACHES, PAINS & CONGESTIONS		
HEAD : HEADACHES / SINUS /NASAL STUFFINESS:		10
CHEST : TIGHTNESS / PHLEGM / WHEEZING-COUGH:		10
ABDOMEN : ACHES / TENDERNESS / GAS / BLOATING:		10

GREASEBALL

SALTY SLIDER

BEANBALL

SCREWBALL

* * HIGH IN CHOLESTEROL
□ MAY CONTAIN CHOLESTEROL
(BUTTER, EGG YOLK)
° MAY RAISE CHOLESTEROL
(SAT. FATS, TRANS FATS)

YOUR PITCHES SCORE: | 120

BASE RUNNING SCORE: | 120

TOTAL PERFORMANCE | 240

283

POST SEASON PLAY:
A NEW YEAR OF FOOD AND FITNESS
COMMITMENT

The results are in: Your progress will continue as the rest of the world gradually realizes how heart disease does not respond as well to high technology as it does to food and fitness changes; and as for cancer, that at least half of today's deaths and disabilities (from heart attacks and cancer) have major personal elements.

Knowing your cholesterol level, then getting it down under 180 and keeping it there will be the essence of effectively protecting yourself from a heart attack.

Reducing your calories from fat and increasing fiber will be the essence of reducing your risk of much cancer.

DISPLAYING YOUR SCOREBOARD

The next two pages are designed to be removed and posted together somewhere that you'll encounter them every day. Perhaps the bathroom mirror, a kitchen cupboard door, an office desk, wherever. Once assembled, they can display a full year of performance.

Effective self-care is outcome-oriented. It targets and measures feeling well and performing fully. It is informed and scientific and it changes important numbers. It takes about five years to change your habits and numbers (and your tissues) in any meaningful way. It's a reconstruction process that takes time. It goes with the grain of your biology rather than cutting across it as do many drugs or technical interventions.

Changes of habit rely on a gradual restoration of numbers, on the natural inclination of biological processes to self-correct to the extent that circumstances are favorable. And that is what the next year is about ... setting a stage of favorable circumstances for what the ancients called "vis medicatrix naturae"; the healing power of nature. Play Ball!

WINNING THE WELLNESS GAME

YOUR SEASON'S PLAY
ScoreBoard™

THE ROOKIES

DRAW LINES BETWEEN THE SAME SYMBOLS FROM MONTH TO MONTH

SCORE SCALE 300	FIRST MONTH	SECOND MONTH	THIRD MONTH	FOURTH MONTH	FIFTH MONTH	SIXTH MONTH
260						
240						
210							Ⓣ
200						
190						
180						
170							Ⓒ
160						
150						
140						
130						
120						
110							Ⓟ
100						
90						
80							Ⓢ
60							Ⓗ

ENTER YOUR STARTING SCORE SYMBOLS HERE.

SYMBOLS ARE IDEAL LEVELS

(left margin, vertically) FOR WALL MOUNT CUT ALONG HERE

287

COACH'S CORNER

FITNESS RISK WARNINGS

Research studies have indicated that cigarette smokers are like overweight individuals, they too are at increased risk of sudden death from unaccustomed physical activity.

Pain is a danger signal. If it occurs during exercise cut back or rest at the first sign of it. Pain says that too much is being asked, that fibers are being torn or that the demand for oxygen is not being met. A weakness has surfaced in the system. Stop hurting yourself and keep your fitness fun.

SEE A PHYSICIAN DURING ANY STAGE OF A
FITNESS PROGRAM
1) if your heart starts jumping or racing

2) if discomfort or pressure occurs in your chest or arms

3) if you experience dizziness or tend to black out

4) if you feel unusually tired as a result of a workout

5) if you develop severe shortness of breath.

288

WINNING THE WELLNESS GAME
POST SEASON PLAY
ScoreBoard™

THE   PROS

CONTINUE TO PLOT YOUR YEAR OF RECORDED PERFORMANCE.

SEVENTH MONTH	EIGHTH MONTH	NINTH MONTH	TENTH MONTH	ELEVENTH MONTH	TWELFTH MONTH	IDEAL RANGE
					300	
					260	
					240	Ⓣ TOT. SCORE
					210	
					200	
					190	
					180	W
					170	
					160	
					150	Ⓒ CHOLESTROL
					140	
					130	W
					120	
					110	Ⓟ PRESSURE
					100	
					90	SUGAR
					80	Ⓢ
					60	Ⓗ HRT. RATE

PASTE PREVIOUS PAGE'S RIGHT EDGE ALONG HERE

FOR WALL MOUNT CUT HERE

289

COACH'S CORNER

A SHORT LIST OF FITNESS BENEFITS

Those who want to keep body weight at optimal levels, remain vigorous into old age, keep blood pressures under control, and avoid heart attacks must begin to start moving around again.

Regular vigorous physical activity has been found to cut the risk of a heart attack in half. There is equally good evidence that it promotes a sense of well-being, tones up muscles, reduces tension and sleeplessness and improves all aspects of the circulation.

Thirty year studies on 16,000 college graduates have confirmed the heart protective effects of regular exercise. It begins with walks that cover five miles a week and is greatest among those who cover about 20 miles a week on foot as a regular habit.

REFERENCES

CANCER

Bailar, J.C. et al. Progress Against Cancer. New Engl. J. of Med. 1986; 314 1226-32.

Bollag, W. Vitamin A And Retinoids: From Nutrition To Pharmacotherapy In Dermatology And Oncology. Lancet, 1983; 2: 860-864.

Carroll, K.K. Dietary Factors In Hormone Dependent Cancers. Current Concepts in Nutrition Vol. 6. Nutrition and Cancer New York John Wiley 1977; 25-40

Committee On Diet, Nutrition and Cancer. National Research Council. Washington D.C. National Academy Press. 1982.

Dormandy, T. L. An Approach To Free Radicals. Lancet. 1983; 2:1010-1014.

Hemekens, C.H. Micro nutrients and cancer prevention. New Engl. J of Med. 1986; 315: 1288-89.

Howe, G.R. et al. Dietary factors and risk of breast cancer: analysis of 12 studies. Journal of the National Cancer Institute. 1990; 82: 561-69.

Jain, M. et al. Dietary factors and risk of lung cancer. International Journal of Cancer. 1990; 45: 287-93.

LaVecchia C, et al. Comparative epidemiology of cancer between the United States and Italy. Cancer Res 1988; 48: 7285-93.

Menkes, M.S., et al. "Serum Beta-Carotene, Vitamins A and E, Selenium and the Risk of Lung Cancer. New Engl. J. of Med. 1986; 315: 1250.

Skrabanek, Petr. False Premises And False Promises Of Breast Cancer Screening. Lancet. 1985; 2: 316-320.

Willett, W. C. et al. Diet and Cancer - an overview. New Engl. J of Med. 1984; 310: 633-38 697-703.

Ziegler, R.G.: A Review Of Epidemiologic Evidence That Carotenoids Reduce The Risk of Cancer. J. Nutr. 1989; 119: 116-122.

FITNESS AND GENERAL HEALTH

Cooper, K.H. The new aerobics. New York NY Evans. 1977.

Koivisto, V. et al: Glycogen depletion during prolonged exercise: influence of glucose, fructose or placebo. J Appl Physiol 1985; 58: 731-37.

Lemon, P.W. et al. Effects of exercise on protein and amino acid metabolism. Medicine and Science In Sports and Exercise. 1981; 13: 141-49.

Manore, M.M. et al. Vitamin B-6 metabolism as affected by exercise in trained and untrained women fed diets differing in carbohydrate and vitamin B-6 content. Am J Clin Nutr 1987; 46: 995-1004.

O'Dea, K. Marked improvements in carbohydrate and lipid metabolism in diabetic Australian Aborigines after temporary revision to traditional lifestyle. Diabetes. 1984; 33: 596-603.

Pietrzik, K. Concept of borderline vitamin deficiencies. Int J Vit Nut Res 1986; (Suppl 1): 61-73.

Rimpala, A.H. et al. Do doctors benefit from their medical knowledge? Lancet 1987; 1:83-86.

Rippe, J.M. et al. Walking for health and fitness. JAMA 1988; 259: 2720-4.

Solomons, N.W. et al. The functional assessment of nutritional status: principles and potential. Nutr Rev. 1983; 41: 33-50.

FOOD SENSITIVITIES

Alun-Jones, V.A. et al. Food intolerance, atopy and irritable bowel syndrome. Lancet. 1964; 2: 1064.

Coello-Ramirez, P. et al. Gastrointestinal occult hemorrhage and gastroduodenitis in cow's milk protein intolerance. J Ped Gastroenterol Nut 1984; 3: 215.

Crook, W.G. The Yeast Connection Jackson, Tennessee: Professional Books, 1985.

Egger, J., et al. "Is Migraine Food Allergy? A Double Blind Controlled Trial of Oligoantigenic Diet Treatment, Lancet. 1984; 2: 719-21.

Fadal, R.G. Introduction to food allergy and other adverse reactions to food. Medical Times. 1989; 60-74.

Hickland, J.A., et al. The Effect of Diet In Rheumatoid Arthritis. Clinical Allergy 1980; 10: 463.

Kremer, Joel M. et al. Fish-Oil Fatty Acid Supplementation In Active Rheumatoid Arthritis. Annals of Internal Med. 1987; 106: 497-502.

Petitpierre, M. et al. Irritable bowel syndrome and hypersensitivity to food. Annals of Allergy 1984; 54: 538-40.

Smith, M.A. et al. Food Intolerance, Atopy and Irritable Bowel Syndrome. Lancet. 1985; 2: 1064.

Woodruff, C.W.: Milk intolerance. Nutr Rev 1976; 34:33.

HEART AND HYPERTENSION

Acheson, R.J. et al. Does consumption of fruit and vegetables protect against stroke? Lancet. 1983; 1: 1191-93.

Anderson, J.W. Dietary fiber, lipids and atherosclerosis. Am J. Cardiol. 1987. 60: 17G-22G.

Barndt, R. et al. Regression and progression of early femeral atheroscorosis in treated hyperlipoproteinemic patients. Annals of Internal Med. 1977; 85: 139-46.

REFERENCES

Blankenhorn, D.H. et al. The influence of diet on the appearance of new lesions in human coronary arteries. JAMA. 1990; 263: 1646-62.

Bonaa, K.H. et al. Effect of fish oils on blood pressure in hypertension. New England Journal of Medicine. 1990; . 322: 795-801.

Brown, J.J. et al. Diet and Hypertension. Lancet. 1984; 2: 671-674.

CASS Investigators. The Coronary Artery Surgery Study: A Randomized Trial of Coronary Artery Bypass Surgery. New Engl. J. Med. 1984; 310: 750-8.

Castelli, W.P. et al. How to help patients cut down on saturated fat: a simple strategy. Postgrad. Med. 1988; 84: 44-56.

Crombie, I.K. et al. Dietary intake of Americans reporting adherence to a low cholesterol diet. American Journal of Public Health. 1990; 698-703.

Enos, W.F. et al. Coronary disease among U.S. soldiers killed in action in Korea. JAMA. 1953; 152: 1090-93.

Final Report of the Subcommittee on Nonpharmacological Therapy of the 1984 Joint National Committee on Detection, Evaluation and Treatment of High Blood Pressure. Hypertension. 1986; 8:5 444-67.

Grobbee, D.E. et al. Does sodium restriction lower the blood pressure? Brit. Med. J. 1986; 293: 27-29.

Grundy, S. M. et al. Influence Of Nicotinic Acid On Metabolism Of Cholesterol and Triglycerides In Man Lipid Research. 1981; 22: 24-36.

Harris, W.S. et al. Fish oils in hypertriglyceridemia: A dose responsive study. American Journal of Clinical Nutrition. 1990; 51: 399-406.

Iso, H. et al: Serum fatty acids and fish intake in rural Japanese, urban Japanese, Japanese American and Caucasian American men. Int J Epidemiology 1989; 18 (2): 374-81.

McCarron, D.A. et al. Nutrition and blood pressure control. Annals of Internal Med. 1983; 98: 697-890.

Mensink, R.P. et al. Effect of dietary transfatty acids on cholesterol levels. New England Journal of Med. 1990; 323: 439-445.

Norris, P.G. et al. Effect of Dietary Supplementation with Fish Oil On Systolic Blood Pressure in Mild Essential Hypertension. Brit. Med. J. 1986; 293: 104.

Ornish, D. et al. Can lifestyle changes reverse coronary heart disease? Lancet. 1990; 1: 129-133.

Report of the National Cholesterol Education Program. Arch. Int. Med. 1988; 148: 36-39.

Rouse, I.L. et al. Blood pressure lowering effect of a vegetarian diet. Lancet. 1983; 1: 5-9.

Shimamoto, T. et al: Trends for coronary heart disease and stroke and their risk factors in Japan. Circulation 1989; 79: 503-15.

Stamler, R. et al. Primary prevention of hypertension by nutritional-hygenic means: final report of a randomized control trial. JAMA. 1989; 262: 1801-7.

Vertes, Victor. Fundamental principles of hypertension: significance and mechanisms. Journal of Cardiology. 1990; 4-9.

Viraq, R. et al. Is impotence an arterial disorder? Lancet. 1985; 1:181-184.

Watts, G.F. et al. Effective lipid lowering diets including lean meat. Br Med J Clin Res 1988; 296: 235-37.

NUTRITION

Cleve, T.L. The Saccharin Disease: Conditions Caused By the Taking of Refined Carbohydrates, Such as Sugar and White Flour. 1978; New Canaan, Connecticut: Keats.

Davis, Clara. Do Young Children Instinctively Know What To Eat? New Engl. J. of Med. 316: 103-106.

Eaton, S. B. et al. Paleolithic nutrition. New Engl. J. Med. 1985; 213: 283-89.

First Health And Nutrition Examination Survey (HANES I). 1971-1974. U.S. Dept. of Health, Education and Welfare, Public Health Service, National Center for Health Statistics. 1979; (PHS 79-1657).

Freudenheim, J.L. et al. Relationships between usual nutrient intake and bone mineral content of women 35-65 years of age. Am. J. Clin. Nutr. 1986; 44: 863-76.

Hallfrisch, J. et al. Mineral Balances of Men and Women Consuming High Fiber Diets. J. Nutr. 1987; 117: 48.

REFERENCES

Health and Human Nutrition Survey, Canadian Dept. of Health, 1975.

Heaton, K.W. Dietary Fiber. Br. Med. J 1990: 300: 1479-80.

Levitt, M.D. et al. Floating stools - flatus versus fat. New Engl. J. Med. 1972; 286: 973-76.

McCulloch, D.K. et al. Influence of imaginative teaching of diet on compliance and metabolic control insulin-dependent diabetes. B.M.J. 1983; 287: 1858-61.

Munier, William B. et al. Intestinal Gas Production-Recent Advances In Flatology. New Engl. J. of Med. 302: 1474-1476.

National Research Council. Recommended Dietary Allowances, 9th ed., National Academy of Sciences, Washington, 1980.

Nationwide Food Consumption Survey, USDA, 1978,

Nationwide food consumption survey 1977-1978. U.S. Dept of Agriculture, Science and Education Administration.

Nutrition and Health. Surgeon General's Report 1988 U.S. Dept. of Health and Human Services.

Small, D.M. et al. Chemistry in the kitchen: making ground meat more healthful. New Engl. J. Med. 1991; 324: 73-7.

Solomons N.W. et al. The Functional assessment of nutritional status: principles and potential. Nutr Rev 1983; 41: 33-50.

Ten State Nutrition Survey, 1968-1970. U.S. Dept of Health, Education and Welfare, Health Services and Mental Health Administration, Center for Disease Control, Atlanta, Georgia. 1972; (HSM 72-8130 through 8134)

Wurtman, R.J. Behavioral effects of nutrients. Lancet. 1983; 1: 1145-47.

STRESS

Benson, H. Your maximum mind. New York, NY Random Hourse 1987.

Case, R.B. Type A behavior and survival after acute myocardial infarction. New Engl. J. Med. 1985; 312: 737-41.

Charlesworth, E.A. et al. Stress Management: A Comprehensive Guide To Wellness. New York, NY: Ballantine, 1984.

Herzog, DB, Copeland, PM. Eating Disorders. N Engl J Med. 1985; 313:295-303.

Moore-Ede, Martin C. et al. The Clocks That Time Us. Harvard University Press. Boston. 1982.

Selye, H. The Stress of LIfe. New York, NY. McGraw-Hill 1978.

WEIGHT

Haber, G.B. et al. Depletion and Disruption of Dietary Fiber. Lancet. 1977; 2: 679-682.

Mirkin, G. Getting Thin. Boston. Little Bown & Co. 1983.

Rizek, R.L. et al. Diets of American Women; 1977 & 1985. Bull Mich Dent Hyg Assoc 1989; 19: 3-6.

GLOSSARY OF TERMS

ADAPTIVE FAILURE: Some degree of loss of the natural capacity of all creatures to maintain a normal steady state such as the blood pressure, blood sugar, body weight etc. Many of today's risk factors are the earliest signs of adaptive failure, signals that the capacity to maintain a normal steady state has been lost to some degree.

ADRENALIN: The body's chemical signal of alarm. Also called epinephrine, it is a hormone made and released from the center of the adrenal gland as well as from certain nerve endings of the automatic nervous system.

ANGIOGRAM: A picture of blood vessels, usually using injected fluids that show up on x-rays.

ANGIOPLASTY: Literally "reshaping blood vessels", but in fact introducing various instruments in an attempt to open clogged or narrowed arteries to greater blood flow.

ANTI-OXIDANT: Any agent, or nutrient (vitamin, mineral or otherwise) that neutralizes the destructive effects of activated oxygen, and thereby has anti-aging and anti-cancer properties.

AORTA: The largest blood vessel coming out of the heart. Its branches serve the entire body.

ARTERIOSCLEROSIS: End stage of the atheroma, when fibrous scar tissue and calcium replace normal elasticity in the adjacent artery wall.

ATHEROMA: A collection of mushy, greasy material (mostly cholesterol) on the innermost wall of arteries, just beneath the inside lining membrane. It projects out into the tunnel of the artery like a tumor, hence the suffix oma. Athero means porridge or gruel or mush.

ATHEROSCLEROSIS: Same as arteriosclerosis, with acknowledgement to the early "mushy tumor".

AUTO-IMMUNITY: Any disorder involving one's own immune system which begins attacking one's own tissues or tissue products causing inflammatory disease and destruction.

BALLOONS: Inflatable cuffs located around tubes that can be inserted into arteries for placement over atheroma deposits to flatten them and partially open arteries.

BETA-BLOCKERS: A family of drugs that block the production of adrenalin (or epinephrine) and its cousin, noradrenalin. Used to control high blood pressure.

BILE: A digestive juice made in the liver, stored in the gall bladder and secreted into the gut during the process of food breakdown and assimilation, especially of fats.

BIOFEEDBACK: A technique of self measurement of such spontaneous natural activities as breathing or sweating or brain waves. They provide indicators to the individual involved of his or her degree of mental control over the process. Biofeedback is a calming strategy for disorders such as stress or migraine headache.

BIOSTRESS: All body manifestations of the fight or flight response to perceived threats. A concept of stress that places equal emphasis on brain and body.

BIPEDAL: Two legged or two footed. An unusual creature in nature, of which we happen to be one example. .

BYPASSING: A vascular surgery option, using veins or arteries to detour blood around narrowed or blocked arteries, usually in the heart; one of today's most common major surgical procedures.

CALCIFICATION: Containing calcium, usually abnormal deposits in body tissues such as arteries.

CAPILLARIES: The tiniest and most numerous of blood vessels in the circulation. They are located as an enormous delivery system network in all tissues connecting the smallest arteries with the smallest veins. Thousands of miles of them.

CARCINOGENS: Agents in the environment, whether food, drink, or atmosphere, that are capable of initiating the cellular changes that can lead to cancer.

CARNITINE: A muscle extract used widely in Europe as an agent for strengthening the heart.

CAROTID ENDARTERECTOMY: Surgical removal of deposits of cholesterol from large arteries of the neck.

CATECHOLOMINES: A collective term for the energizing and heat-producing hormones epinephrine and norepinephrine.

CELLULOSE GUM: A plant fiber with viscous or gummy physical properties. Captures cholesterol.

CENTRIFUGATION: Spinning a liquid to separate out its components.

CHELATION: A biochemical infusion technique for capturing certain metals in tissues, as for example calcium in hardened arteries. After more than 40 years of claims and tests, still not of proven clinical benefit.

CHOLESTEROL: An essential building block of all body tissues, a chemical fat of structural stability which toughens structures. Essential to life in normal amounts, when present in excess it accumulates to produce toxic effects in all tissues, especially the arteries.

CHOLESTYRAMINE: A non digestible drug that captures cholesterol in the gut, thereby lowering its levels in the blood.

CLEAN FOOD: Dietary items that contain little or no fat. See also DIRTY FOOD.

CORONARY ARTERY DISEASE: All degrees of heart artery narrowing beginning with the earliest deposits of cholesterol in artery walls. (In our culture, that's late in childhood.)

DEFIBRILLATOR: A machine that provides electrical interventions to restore a normal heart beat.

DEMAND-PERFORMANCE CURVE: A 2-dimensional plot expressing the relationship between a progressive load and tissue response; an engineering device for better understanding of how input excesses contribute to the moods of overload and stress. (Its use enables a better analysis of stress for prevention and control).

311

DILATATION: An opening up, as with the pupil of the eye in low light.

DIRTY FOOD: Dietary items that contain too much fat, say more than 20% of its calories.

DIURETIC: An agent that promotes urine formation.

DIVERTICULITIS: Inflammation of tiny outpouchings of large bowel or colon wall at the lowest levels of the digestive tract. They occur in response to years of high colon pressures from a chronically under fibered diet.

DYSRHYTHMIA: A disordered heart beat: too fast, too slow or irregular.

EMULSIFY: To disperse into a solution, as soap does grease.

ENDORPHINS: Chemicals produced by tissues in the body that produce a pleasant feeling in the brain.

ENZYMES: Chemical agents of change that produce predetermined chemical outcomes or products.

ESSENTIAL FATTY ACIDS: Basic fats that we all need but cannot make on our own. They must be present in the diet, as in nuts, grains, vegetables, and whole grain flour products. Eating whole foods is the alternative to cooking with them or adding them as salad oils.

ESSENTIAL HYPERTENSION: An elevated blood pressure for which no explanation (such as kidney or artery disease) can be found.

FIBER: Indigestible constituents of a normal dietary item, almost always of plant origin. There are hundreds of them.

FOOD ENCOUNTER: A modern meal for weight control, consisting of low fat, high fiber foods in limited amounts from a limited selection.

FRAMINGHAM STUDY: A long-term scientific evaluation of the health outcomes of a population in a small New England city. It has helped establish risk factors for heart attacks.

FREE RADICALS: Extremely irritating and very short-lived products of normal body chemistry. They are capable of promoting tissue injury, aging and cancer.

GASTRO-ENTERITIS: An inflamed or irritated digestive tract.

GLYCEROL: Half a sugar molecule, and a source of energy, used as a building block for body fat.

GUAR GUM: A plant fiber with mucinous or gummy properties, used extensively in the food processing industry. Lowers cholesterol.

HEPATITIS: An inflamed liver, usually from a virus infection or from chemical irritation.

HISTAMINE: A chemical released by many tissues in the body especially when they are allergic to something and reacting to it.

HOMEOSTATIC: A steady state in the body such as the blood pressure level or sugar level resulting from a balance of natural opposing forces, some tending to raise it and others to lower it.

HOSTILITY COMPLEX: Any collection of angry responses to a perceived threat. Part of stress.

HOT SPOTS: A runner's term for small, tender points of injury in the muscles, ligiments or tendons.

HYDROGENATION: The addition of hydrogen atoms to a molecule, usually to a fat molecule to saturate it by loading up all its available chemical linkages.

HYPERCHOLESTEROLEMIA: High cholesterol blood levels.

HYPERLIPIDEMIA: High fat levels in the blood, cholesterol and or triglyceride.

HYPERTENSION: High blood pressure.

INSULIN: A hormone made in the pancreas that helps keep the blood sugar normal. It is a hormone that serves as a feeding signal to the tissues of the body.

ISCHEMIA: Oxygen deprived, usually the result of a poor circulation.

LASERS: Intense beams of heat from spectrum-narrowed light, used medically to produce controlled burning or scarring.

LECITHIN: An emulsifying agent found throughout nature, and promoted commercially to lower the blood cholesterol.

LIFE EXPECTANCY: The statistical age at which the average newborn individual in a given culture can expect to die.

LIFE SPAN: The age at which the average member of any species dies, in the absence of disease or injury. In the human, it appears to be 100 years with a range of 80 to 120.

LINOLEIC ACID: An essential fatty acid, present in many grains and seeds and vegetables.

MAGNESIUM: A metallic element in the diet that is essential to health. Sometimes used as a food supplement for its calming effect.

MAXEPA: Trade name for a source of omega-3 ocean fish oil.

MELANOMA: A potentially lethal pigmented tumor, usually of the skin.

MUCIN-GELATIN FIBERS: Indigestible food elements with mucus-like physical properties that often are able to lower the blood cholesterol.

MULTI-FACTORAL: More than one contributing cause.

NEUROTRANSMITTER: A chemical that enables individual nerves to stimulate and thus to signal each other.

NEW BRAIN: The cauliflower like top half of our brain that makes us intelligent and human. Also called neo cortex.

NIACIN: One of the B vitamins. In large amounts it has a cholesterol-lowering effect.

NIBBLING FOODSTYLE: Eating patterns that emphasize small, frequent food encounters of a low fat, high fiber composition.

NICOTINIC ACID: A chemical variant of niacin, the B vitamin.

NITROGLYCERINE: A medication that helps open up narrowed coronary arteries.

NORADRENALIN: A neurotransmitter chemical made in the adrenal glands and in the automatic nervous system.

NORMAL DISTRIBUTION CURVE: The graphic pattern created whenever a large population of numbers can be shown to cluster above and below an average number.

OAT BRAN : A grain fiber with gummy properties that can capture cholesterol.

OLD BRAIN: The hidden, older, bottom half of the brain, also called the thalamus and hypothalamus. It's the engine room of the body; the monitoring system of all body functions, and we share its structures and chemicals with many other creatures.

OMEGA-3: A chemical designation of the active element in fish oils.

OSTEOPOROSIS: Thin, fragile bones, often complicating the lives of older women. Its most dangerous outcomes are fractured hips.

OXIDATION: A chemical process wherein oxygen links up with other chemical components in a generally irreversible way.

OXYGENATION: Same as the above, but in a more reversible way.

PANCREATITIS: An irritated or inflamed pancreas.

PECTINS: A fruit fiber with gummy properties that can capture cholesterol.

PERFUSION: The irrigation of tissues along normal blood vessel channels.

PHOSPHOLIPIDS: Special fats containing a phosphate group.

PLATELET: The smallest blood cell in the circulation, of which there are thousands in every drop. They are circulating emergency vehicles ready to shatter upon encountering a break in the lining of blood vessels to release agents that cause the blood to clot and inflammation to start.

POLYUNSATURATED: A chemical description of the linkages between the carbon molecules in a fat. They are several in number (poly) and capable of taking up more hydrogen (unsaturated).

POTASSIUM: An essential mineral nutrient present in all fruits and vegetables. It's levels are declining in our diet, and aggravating the blood pressure effects of the sodium excesses in our diet.

PROSTAGLANDINS: A family of natural chemicals produced by the body's tissues to achieve a local effect on blood clotting or blood vessel behavior.

PSYLLIUM: A gummy fiber isolated from the seed of a plant from India, used as a laxative. Lowers cholesterol.

REBOUNDER: A small trampoline, useful in producing and maintaining fitness in an office, by a computer terminal, or in a home setting.

RISK FACTOR: Any element in one's habits or numbers that increase the risk of premature death.

RULE OF FIVES: A shorthand reminder of the essential practices of a low fat/high fiber foodstyle.

SACCHARINE: One of the earliest of the non-caloric sugar substitutes.

SATURATED: A chemical term describing totally occupied linkages between the carbon atoms of a fat molecule. No more hydrogen can be taken up.

SERUM LEVELS: Measurements of circulating elements in the blood after all red cells have been removed by allowing the blood to clot.

SHAVERS: Surgical instruments that scrape or slice cholesterol deposits from artery walls.

STENOSIS: A narrowing of some major part of the circulation.

STENTS: Tiny tubes that are inserted permanently into arteries as tunneling devices through blockages.

STOP-IT: A mnemonic device for reminding you of the many strategies possible in biostress management.

STUTTERING STROKES: Transient and often progressive episodes of paralysis of an arm or leg. Transient speech or memory loss.

TACHYCARDIA: A fast heart rate.

TERMINAL ILIUM: The end part of the small intestine just before it enters the large intestine or colon.

TISSUE TURNOVER: The natural replacement process of all components of all structures of all cells in the body. It is continuous and constant throughout life.

TOCOPHEROL: Chemical name for the fat soluble anti-oxidant vitamin E.

TRANS FATTY ACIDS: Twisted fat molecules that result from the high temperatures and pressures of modern processing. They do not occur in nature and in excess can promote elevated cholesterol levels and other problems.

TRIGLYCERIDES: Chemical term for the most common kind of fat. It is the fat of obesity. It can circulate in elevated levels in the blood and, like cholesterol, it can narrow arteries.

TYPE A VS. TYPE B PERSONALITIES: Shorthand for personality types, A tending to be energetically aggressive and leading, B tending to be relaxed, cool and following.

UNSATURATED: Chemical term describing available linkages for hydrogen between the carbon atoms of a fat molecule.

VITAMIN E: A fat soluble anti-oxidant vitamin.

WALKING WOUNDED: Usually symptomless individuals with demonstrable risk factors. They often function with medication, over-the-counter and prescribed.

WHEAT BRAN: A laxative fiber from wheat that bulks the stool by holding 9 times its weight in water. A good laxative with little or no effect on cholesterol.

XANTHUM: A food fiber with gummy properties that can capture cholesterol and lower blood levels.

INDEX

PERSONAL
ACTION NOTES

PERSONAL
ACTION NOTES

PERSONAL
ACTION NOTES

PERSONAL ACTION NOTES

PERSONAL
ACTION NOTES

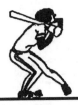

PERSONAL
ACTION NOTES